JARVIS

Mental Health in the Medical Setting: Delivery, Workforce Needs, and Emerging Best Practices

Editor

PETER F. BUCKLEY

PSYCHIATRIC CLINICS OF NORTH AMERICA

www.psych.theclinics.com

March 2015 • Volume 38 • Number 1

ELSEVIER

1600 John F. Kennedy Boulevard • Suite 1800 • Philadelphia, Pennsylvania, 19103-2899

http://www.theclinics.com

PSYCHIATRIC CLINICS OF NORTH AMERICA Volume 38, Number 1
March 2015 ISSN 0193-953X, ISBN-13: 978-0-323-39141-2

Editor: Joanne Husovski
Developmental Editor: Stephanie Carter

Psychiatric Clinics of North America (ISSN 0193-953X) is published quarterly by Elsevier Inc., 360 Park Avenue South, New York, NY 10010-1710. Months of issue are March, June, September, and December. Business and Editorial Offices: 1600 John F. Kennedy Blvd., Suite 1800, Philadelphia, PA 19103-2899. Periodicals postage paid at New York, NY and additional mailing offices. Subscription prices are $300.00 per year (US individuals), $546.00 per year (US institutions), $150.00 per year (US students/residents), $365.00 per year (Canadian individuals), $455.00 per year (international individuals), $687.00 per year (Canadian & international institutions), and $220.00 per year (Canadian & international students/residents). Foreign air speed delivery is included in all *Clinics*' subscription prices. All prices are subject to change without notice. **POSTMASTER:** Send address changes to *Psychiatric Clinics of North America*, Elsevier Health Sciences Division, Subscription Customer Service, 3251 Riverport Lane, Maryland Heights, MO 63043. Customer Service: 1-800-654-2452 (US). From outside the United States, call 1-314-447-8871. Fax: 1-314-447-8029. E-mail: journalscustomerservice-usa@elsevier.com (for print support) and journalsonlinesupport-usa@elsevier.com (for online support).

Reprints. For copies of 100 or more, of articles in this publication, please contact the Commercial Reprints Department, Elsevier Inc., 360 Park Avenue South, New York, New York 10010-1710. Tel.: 212-633-3874, Fax: 212-633-3820, E-mail: reprints@elsevier.com.

Psychiatric Clinics of North America is covered in *MEDLINE/PubMed (Index Medicus)*, *Current Contents/Social and Behavioral Sciences, Social Science Citation Index, Embase/Excerpta Medica,* and PsycINFO.

Printed in the United States of America.

Contributors

EDITOR

PETER F. BUCKLEY, MD
Dean, Medical College of Georgia; Professor, Department of Psychiatry and Health Behavior, Georgia Regents University, Augusta, Georgia

AUTHORS

MICHAEL A. AMBROSE, BA
Division of Behavioral and Developmental Health, Department of Pediatrics, Mount Sinai Medical Center, New York, New York

RONEN ARNON ANNUNZIATO, PhD
Assistant Professor, Division of Behavioral and Developmental Health, Department of Pediatrics, Mount Sinai Medical Center, New York; Department of Psychology, Fordham University, Bronx, New York

CHRISTINE BARNEY, MD
Independent Practitioner, White River Junction, Vermont

ABIR K. BEKHET, PhD, RN, HSMI
Assistant Professor of Psychiatric and Mental Health Nursing, Marquette University College of Nursing, Milwaukee, Wisconsin

KELLEY CHUANG, MA
Division of Behavioral and Developmental Health, Department of Pediatrics, Mount Sinai Medical Center, New York, New York

AMANDA L. COX, MD
Assistant Professor, Division of Pediatric Allergy and Immunology, Mount Sinai Medical Center, New York, New York

ANITA DEMPSEY, PhD, APRN, PMHCNS-BC
Associate Director, Psychiatric and Mental Health Nurse Practitioner Program in the Wright State University–Miami Valley College of Nursing and Health; Assistant Professor of Nursing, College of Nursing and Health, Wright State University, Dayton, Ohio

D. EDWARD DENEKE, MD
Assistant Director of Resident Education, Department of Psychiatry, University of Michigan Health System, University of Michigan, Ann Arbor, Michigan

THOMAS E. FLUENT, MD
Clinical Assistant Professor, Department of Psychiatry, University of Michigan Health System, University of Michigan, Ann Arbor, Michigan

SANDRA L. FRITSCH, MD
Training Director, Child and Adolescent Psychiatry; Department of Psychiatry, Maine
Medical Center; Associate Clinical Professor, Tufts University School of Medicine,
Portland, Maine

RAMONA O. HOPKINS, PhD
Department of Psychology and Neuroscience Center, Brigham Young University, Provo,
Utah; Division of Pulmonary and Critical Care, Department of Medicine, Intermountain
Medical Center, Murray, Utah

JAMES C. JACKSON, PsyD
Center for Health Services Research, Vanderbilt University Medical Center, Vanderbilt
University School of Medicine, Nashville, Tennessee; VA-Tennessee Valley Health
System (VA-TVHS), Murfreesboro, Tennessee

NATHANIEL MITCHELL, PhD
Department of Psychology, Spalding University, Louisville, Kentucky

JENNIFER MOYE, PhD
Director, Geriatric Mental Health, VA Boston Health Care System; Associate Professor,
Department of Psychiatry, Harvard Medical School, Boston, Massachusetts

CHLOE MULLARKEY, BS
Division of Behavioral and Developmental Health, Department of Pediatrics, Mount Sinai
Medical Center, New York, New York

SIRISHA NARAYANA, MD
Assistant Professor, Department of Medicine, UCSF School of Medicine, San Francisco,
California

MARK W. OVERTON, MD
Psychiatrist, Northern Maine Medical Center, Fort Kent, Maine

NOGA L. RAVID, BA
Mount Sinai School of Medicine, New York, New York

JUDY RIBAK, PhD, APRN, PMHCNS-BC
Assistant Professor of Nursing, Wright State University, College of Nursing and Health,
Dayton, Ohio

DOUGLAS R. ROBBINS, MD
Division Chief, Child and Adolescent Psychiatry, Maine Medical Center; Chair, The
Glickman Family Center for Child and Adolescent Psychiatry; Clinical Professor, Tufts
University School of Medicine, Portland, Maine

SUSAN J. ROUSE, PMH-CNS-BC
VA Boston Health Care System, Boston, Massachusetts

COLLEEN M. RYAN, MD
Staff Surgeon, Department of Surgery, Massachusetts General Hospital, Harvard Medical
School, Boston Massachusetts

JEFFREY C. SCHNEIDER, MD
Department of Physical Medicine and Rehabilitation, Spaulding Rehabilitation Hospital,
Harvard Medical School, Boston, Massachusetts

HEATHER E. SCHULTZ, MD, MPH
Clinical Instructor, Inpatient Psychiatry, University of Michigan Health System, University of Michigan, Ann Arbor, Michigan

SHAWN CHRISTOPHER SHEA, MD
Director, Training Institute for Suicide Assessment and Clinical Interviewing (TISA), Newbury, New Hampshire

EYAL SHEMESH, MD
Associate Professor, Division of Behavioral and Developmental Health, Department of Pediatrics, Mount Sinai Medical Center, New York, New York

SCOTT H. SICHERER, MD
Professor, Division of Pediatric Allergy and Immunology, Mount Sinai Medical Center, New York, New York

FREDERICK J. STODDARD Jr, MD
Department of Psychiatry, Massachusetts General Hospital, Harvard Medical School, Boston, Massachusetts

M. JANE SURESKY, DNP, PMHCNS-BC
Assistant Professor of Psychiatric and Mental Health Nursing, Frances Payne Bolton School of Nursing, Case Western Reserve University, Cleveland, Ohio

CHRISTOPHER J. WONG, MD
Assistant Professor, Division of General Internal Medicine, Department of Medicine, University of Washington, Seattle, Washington

JACLENE A. ZAUSZNIEWSKI, PhD, RN-BC, FAAN
Kate Hanna Harvey Professor of Community Health Nursing, Frances Payne Bolton School of Nursing, Case Western Reserve University, Cleveland, Ohio

Contents

> Depression and anxiety disorders are common conditions with significant morbidity. Many screening tools of varying length have been well validated for these conditions in the office-based setting. Novel instruments, including Internet-based and computerized adaptive testing, may be promising tools in the future. The best evidence for cost-effectiveness currently is for screening of major depression linked with the collaborative care model for treatment. Data are not conclusive regarding comparative cost-effectiveness of screening for multiple conditions at once or for other conditions. This article reviews screening tools for depression and anxiety disorders in the ambulatory setting.

> Despite strong efforts, the diagnosis and treatment of depression bring many challenges in the primary care setting. Screening for depression has been shown to be effective only if reliable systems of care are in place to ensure appropriate treatment by clinicians and adherence by patients. New evidence-based models of care for depression exist, but spread has been slow because of inadequate funding structures and conflicts within current clinical culture. The Affordable Care Act introduces potential opportunities to reorganize funding structures, conceivably leading to increased adoption of these collaborative care models. Suicide screening remains controversial.

> Most older patients adapt after catastrophic medical diagnoses and treatments, but a significant number may develop posttraumatic stress disorder (PTSD) symptoms. PTSD symptoms create added burden for the individual, family, and health care system for the patient's recovery. Medical-related PTSD may be underdiagnosed by providers who may be unaware that these health problems can lead to PTSD symptoms. Treatment research is lacking, but pharmacologic and nonpharmacologic approaches to treatment may be extrapolated and adjusted from the literature focusing on younger adults. Additional study is needed.

Diabetes mellitus is a common childhood illness, and its management is often complicated by mental health challenges. Psychiatric comorbidities are common, including anxiety, depression, and eating disorders. The illness can profoundly affect the developing brain and family functioning and have lifelong consequences. The child mental health provider can provide valuable assistance to support the child and family and assessment and treatment of comorbid mental health problems and to promote positive family functioning and normal developmental progress.

As food allergy increases, more research is devoted to its influence on patient and family mental health and quality of life (QoL). This article discusses the effects on parent and child QoL, as well as distress, while appraising the limitations of knowledge given the methods used. Topics include whether QoL and distress are affected compared with other illnesses, assessment of distress and QoL in parents compared with children, concerns about food allergy-related bullying, and the necessity for evidence-based interventions. Suggestions are offered for how to improve QoL and reduce distress on the way to better coping with food allergy.

Critical illness can and often does lead to significant cognitive impairment and to the development of psychological disorders. These conditions are persistent and, although they improve with time, often fail to completely abate. Although the functional correlates of cognitive and psychological morbidity (depression, anxiety, and posttraumatic stress disorder) have been studied, they may include poor quality of life, inability to return to work or to work at previously established levels, and inability to function effectively in emotional and interpersonal domains. The potential etiologies of cognitive impairment and psychological morbidity in ICU survivors are particularly poorly understood and may vary widely across patients. Potential contributors may include the potentially toxic effects of sedatives and narcotics, delirium, hypoxia, glucose dysregulation, metabolic derangements, and inflammation. Patients with preexisting vulnerabilities, including predisposing genetic factors, and frail elderly populations may be at particular risk for emergence of acceleration of conditions such as mild cognitive impairment.

Burn injuries pose complex biopsychosocial challenges to recovery and improved comprehensive care. The physical and emotional sequelae of burns differ, depending on burn severity, individual resilience, and stage of development when they occur. Most burn survivors are resilient and recover, whereas some are more vulnerable and have complicated outcomes. Physical rehabilitation is affected by orthopedic, neurologic, and metabolic complications and disabilities. Psychiatric recovery is affected by pain, mental disorders, substance abuse, and burn stigmatization. Individual resilience, social supports, and educational or occupational achievements affect outcomes.

Anita Dempsey and Judy Ribak

The role of the psychiatric mental health clinical nurse specialist (PMHCNS) is now in a precarious position. At first glance, some may say it is on the verge of extinction. In this article, a brief history of the role of the PMHCNS is reviewed along with current education, practice, role, and American Nurses Credentialing Center certification of the PMHCNS. The future implications and considerations of the unique functions of the PMHCNS for an advanced practice registered nurse with a psychiatric mental health specialization are discussed.

Jaclene A. Zauszniewski, Abir K. Bekhet, and M. Jane Suresky

This integrative review summarizes current research on resilience in adult family members who have a relative with a diagnosed mental disorder considered serious. Within the context of resilience theory, studies identifying risk/vulnerability and positive/protective factors in family members are summarized, and studies examining 7 indicators of resilience, including acceptance, hardiness, hope, mastery, self-efficacy, sense of coherence, and resourcefulness, are described. Implications for clinical practice and recommendations for future research are presented.

Special Article

Shawn Christopher Shea and Christine Barney

This article provides a useful introduction to the art of role-playing in both the individual format and the group format using scripted group role-playing (SGRP). Role-playing can provide powerful learning opportunities, but to do so it must be done well. This article imparts guidance toward this goal. SGRP may greatly enhance the acquisition of critical complex interviewing skills, such as suicide assessment and uncovering domestic violence, in health care providers across all disciplines, an educational goal that has not been achievable to date. Although research is at an early stage of development, the hope represented by SGRP is tangible.

PSYCHIATRIC CLINICS OF NORTH AMERICA

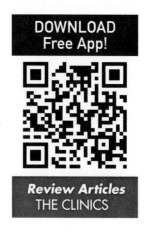

Preface

Mental Health in the Medical Setting: Service Delivery, Workforce Needs, and Emerging Best Practices

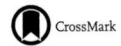

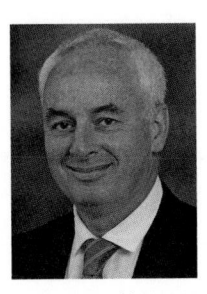

Peter F. Buckley, MD
Editor

Few topics, if any, in mental health attract such widespread and sustained interest as the issue of the interface and commonality between physical and mental illness. Through the stellar contributions of the authors herein, this issue addresses important and topical aspects relating to this interface.

Mental illnesses do not occur in a vacuum. Physical health and mental health are inextricably linked. Moreover, as the biology of mental illnesses is gradually, and hopefully inexorably, being elucidated, the overlap between physical illnesses and mental illnesses has become even more apparent. This dualism is further underscored most recently in the political arena, with implementation of the Affordable Care Act in the United States, which will likely, and certainly hopefully, promote greater congruence and overlap between service provision for both physical and psychiatric conditions.

These observations "set the stage" for readers of this issue of *Psychiatric Clinics of North America*. Clearly, bioterrorism is now a major consideration in all areas of society and also requires us, as clinicians, to be ever prepared and vigilant. It is apt, then, that we begin this issue of *Psychiatric Clinics of North America* with a terrific article on emergency mental health support to individuals who are caught up in bioterrorism. Subsequent articles focus on other salient physical conditions that pose particular challenges to mental health: burns, prolonged stay in the intensive care unit, comorbidities in the elderly, food allergies, depression and other common primary care conditions, and childhood diabetes. This issue also addresses some of the cardinal issues of evidence-based practices, interviewing for practices, the expanding role for nurses (in both mental and physical aspects of health care), and the power of healing that supportive family members bring as members of the multidisciplinary team.

Psychiatr Clin N Am 38 (2015) xi–xii
http://dx.doi.org/10.1016/j.psc.2014.11.010
0193-953X/15/$ – see front matter © 2015 Elsevier Inc. All rights reserved.

psych.theclinics.com

All in all, these articles are an interesting and representative sample of the many areas of interface between physical and mental illnesses. The authors deserve our thanks for their stellar contributions.

I hope that you enjoy this issue of *Psychiatry Clinics of North America*.

Peter F. Buckley, MD
Medical College of Georgia
Georgia Regents University
1120 15th Street, AA-1002
Augusta, GA 30912, USA

E-mail address:
PBuckley@gru.edu

Office-Based Screening of Common Psychiatric Conditions

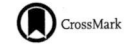 CrossMark

Sirisha Narayana, MD[a], Christopher J. Wong, MD[b],*

KEYWORDS

- Screening • Depression • Anxiety • Cost-effectiveness • Outcomes

KEY POINTS

- Depression and anxiety disorders are common and significant conditions in the general population.
- Multiple well-validated screening instruments exist, which may be easily administered in an outpatient setting. These include the Patient Health Questionnaire (PHQ)-9 for depression, the Generalized Anxiety Disorder (GAD)-7 for anxiety disorders, and the Primary Care–Posttraumatic Stress Disorder Screen (PC-PTSD) for PTSD.
- Despite the availability of screening tools, the overall cost-effectiveness of general screening for anxiety or depression is uncertain.
- Screening for depression is recommended by some preventive health guidelines, and is most likely cost-effective in the setting of high prevalence and the availability of treatment using a collaborative care model.

INTRODUCTION

Depression and anxiety disorders are common and significantly affect health worldwide. Treatment options including psychotherapy and pharmacotherapy have expanded and in many regions are easily accessible. Yet these disorders may be undertreated. Approximately 40% of patients screening positive for anxiety disorders were not receiving treatment in one study, and patients with depression were being treated only 50% of the time in another study, with disparities among ethnic/racial groups.[1,2] Screening is therefore an important element to consider in the effort to reduce the overall burden of depression and anxiety disorders. Multiple screening modalities have been

This article first appeared in Med Clin N Am 2014;98(5):959–980.
Funding sources: None.
Conflicts of interest: None.
[a] Department of Medicine, UCSF School of Medicine, 533 Parnassus Avenue, UC Hall, San Francisco, CA 94143, USA; [b] Division of General Internal Medicine, Department of Medicine, University of Washington, 4245 Roosevelt Way Northeast, Box 354760, Seattle, WA 98105, USA
* Corresponding author.
E-mail address: cjwong@uw.edu

developed to facilitate diagnosis and treatment of common mental health disorders in the primary care setting. With the many options available, it is important to have an understanding of the strengths and limitations of these tools, the recommendations from major guidelines regarding screening, and where unanswered questions remain.

SCREENING ASYMPTOMATIC PATIENTS FOR PSYCHIATRIC CONDITIONS—GENERAL CONSIDERATIONS

Screening requires several conditions be present to be considered effective (**Table 1**).[3] First, the illness should be significantly burdensome in the population to warrant screening. The reported prevalence of depression and anxiety disorders is high, although estimates vary by location, classification, and duration (**Table 2** shows selected studies). Prevalence estimates should be interpreted with caution. Variations exist by country,[4] and because patients with psychiatric disorders may incur more physician visits, clinic-based point prevalence estimates are generally higher than those using population-based methods (eg, generalized anxiety disorder had a 3.1% prevalence in a community sample vs 7.6% in a clinic-based sample).[1,5] Second, a highly sensitive and specific screening test that is easy to administer must exist. Third, the illness should be identified by screening at a treatable stage or a stage in which early treatment is more effective than later treatment. The concept of early treatment is more complex with psychiatric illnesses: by definition patients are symptomatic, but the natural history of common psychiatric conditions is varied; they may have potentially lifelong

Table 1 Conceptual framework for psychiatric disease screening		
Criteria	**Nonpsychiatry Examples**	**Comparison with Psychiatric Disease Screening**
Condition causes significant burden in the population	Rare but severe: phenylketonuria in newborns Common and causing morbidity: diabetes, hypertension	Similar to diabetes and hypertension, depression and anxiety disorders are common (see **Table 2**) and cause substantial morbidity
An easy-to-administer, effective screening test exists	Blood pressure Fasting glucose or A1c	Screening tools are readily available, generally consist of questionnaires
Early treatment is more effective than later treatment	Cancer screening: goal is to identify disease at an earlier stage at which treatment is more effective Diabetes: goal is to identify disease before it is symptomatic to initiate treatment and prevent complications	In contrast, by definition there is no asymptomatic stage for depression and anxiety disorders Varied natural history: waxing/waning, episodic/self-limited, lifelong
Benefits of screening tests and subsequent treatment outweigh potential harms, at acceptable cost	Mammography: Harms include radiation, follow-up imaging, biopsies, worry. Optimal target population and interval still debated	Harms of screening tools themselves generally minimal; harms and costs are associated with subsequent treatment

Table 2
Prevalence of common psychiatric disorders

	12-mo Prevalence[5] (%)	Lifetime Prevalence[8] (%)
Any mood disorder[a]	9.5	20.8
Major depressive disorder	6.7	16.6
Any anxiety disorder[b]	18.1	28.8
Generalized anxiety disorder	3.1	5.7
PTSD	3.5	6.8
ADHD	4.1	8.1

Abbreviation: ADHD, attention-deficit and hyperactivity disorder.

[a] Includes major depressive disorder, dysthymia, and bipolar I and II disorders.

[b] Includes panic disorder, agoraphobia without panic, specific phobia, social phobia, generalized anxiety disorder, obsessive-compulsive disorder, separation anxiety disorder. Posttraumatic stress disorder subtracted from the published total because it is now classified as a trauma- and stressor-related disorder.

conditions such as generalized anxiety disorder, with waxing and waning severity, or episodic with a self-limited course as with major depressive disorder. Fourth, the screening tests and treatment must have clinically meaningful benefits that outweigh potential harms to a patient at an acceptable cost to society. For the purposes of this review, the third and fourth criteria are considered together as general effectiveness.

Case Definitions

Unless specified otherwise, this review discusses screening tools validated against structured diagnostic interviews. Most of the tools described later were tested against the Diagnostic and Statistical Manual of Mental Disorders (DSM)-III, the DSM-IV, or World Health Organization (WHO) definitions. The newer DMS-V diagnostic criteria for a major depressive episode and generalized anxiety disorder have only minor differences compared with those of DSM-IV, not expected to substantially affect the performance of these measures.[6,7]

DEPRESSION
Burden of Disease

The 12-month prevalence of major depressive disorder in the United States is estimated at 6.7%, and the lifetime prevalence of any mood disorder is approximately 20%.[5,8] Depression is estimated as the fourth leading cause of disability adjusted life years worldwide.[4]

Screening Tools

General population
Many screening tools exist for depressive disorders (**Table 3**). Selected tools are discussed below.

PHQ-9 and PHQ-2 The PHQ-9 evolved from the full Primary Care Evaluation of Mental Disorders (PRIME-MD) instrument developed in the early 1990s to diagnose depression, anxiety, somatoform disorder, and alcohol and eating disorders.[9] The PRIME-MD necessitated significant investment of physician-patient time (>11 minutes) and led to the shorter PHQ,[10] and subsequently the PHQ-9, the 9-item depression module from the full PHQ (**Box 1**). It is scored 0 to 27, with a score of 10 or more indicating a possible depressive disorder. Scores of 5, 10, 15, and 20 represented mild, moderate,

Table 3
Selected tools and considerations for depression screening

Population	Tools	Description
General population/primary care	PHQ-9 PHQ-2 Others	PHQ-9 and PHQ-2 freely available Screening recommended by USPSTF if treatment resources available
Veterans	PHQ-9 PHQ-2	The Veterans Affairs administration recommends yearly screening of veterans for depression using the PHQ-2[66] with follow-up as needed with PHQ-9 and a full assessment; and those at higher risk of developing depression (patients with hepatitis C beginning interferon treatment or patients post-MI) be given the PHQ-9 when depression is suspected Use caution in screening patients older than 75 y because instruments may not perform as well as between the ages of 65 and 75 y[67]
Medical comorbidities	Various, including PHQ-9, PHQ-2, HADS, BDI, Montgomery and Asberg Depression Rating Scale, others	Increased rates of depression in patients with central nervous system disease, cardiovascular disease, and malignancy[68–71] Up to 20% of patients with myocardial infarction meet DSM-IV criteria for major depression. The American Heart Association advocates for screening for depression after MI. Approximately half of post-MI depression resolves without treatment. Some evidence of treatment efficacy in patients poststroke, post-MI[68–75] The PHQ-9 and HADS have been studied in patients with coronary disease and are comparable in effectiveness for screening[76] The PHQ-9 has been used in multiple medical settings, including rheumatology, ophthalmology, and spinal cord injury[77]
Elderly	PHQ-9 PHQ-2 GDS	GDS score >5: sensitivity 0.92, specificity 0.81 for major depression
Addiction	PHQ-9, others	Consider screening in patients with substance use disorders
Psychiatric comorbidities	PHQ-9, others	Consider screening in patients with other psychiatric conditions, including anxiety disorders and PTSD

Abbreviations: GDS, Geriatric Depression Scale; HADS, Hospital Anxiety and Depression Scale; MI, myocardial infarction.

Box 1
Patient health questionnaire-9

Over the Last 2 wk, How Often Have You Been Bothered by Any of the Following Problems?	Not At all	Several Days	More Than Half the Days	Nearly Every Day
1. Little interest or pleasure in doing things	0	1	2	3
2. Feeling down, depressed, or hopeless	0	1	2	3
3. Trouble falling or staying asleep, or sleeping too much	0	1	2	3
4. Feeling tired or having little energy	0	1	2	3
5. Poor appetite or overeating	0	1	2	3
6. Feeling bad about yourself — or that you are a failure or have let yourself or your family down	0	1	2	3
7. Trouble concentrating on things, such as reading the newspaper or watching television	0	1	2	3
8. Moving or speaking so slowly that other people could have noticed? Or the opposite — being so fidgety or restless that you have been moving around a lot more than usual	0	1	2	3
9. Thoughts that you would be better off dead or of hurting yourself in some way	0	1	2	3
	0 +	_____ +	_____ +	_____
			=Total Score:	_____

If you checked off any problems, how difficult have these problems made it for you to do your work, take care of things at home, or get along with other people?

Not difficult at all   Somewhat difficult   Very difficult   Extremely difficult

From The Patient Health Questionnaire (PHQ) Screeners. Available at: http://www. phqscreeners.com/overview.aspx?Screener=02_PHQ-9. Accessed May 1, 2014.

moderately severe, and severe depression, respectively. To make the diagnosis of major depression, at least one of the first two questions must score a two or greater; this includes anhedonia and feelings of low mood/depression. The PHQ-9 module aligns closely with the DSM-IV diagnosis of depression and accordingly includes a question of whether symptoms impair functioning. At a cutoff score of 10, the PHQ-9 was found to have 0.88 sensitivity and specificity, and a likelihood ratio of 7.1, in the population studied (mean age 30–40 years, mostly white women with few medical comorbidities).[11] The validity of the PHQ-9 has been further demonstrated in a general population.[12] Subsequent meta-analyses confirmed high sensitivity of the PHQ-9, although one study did demonstrate a lower specificity of 0.77, possibly due to a lower prevalence of depression in the population studied.[13] Despite the heterogeneity of the studies in terms of settings (community, primary care, and hospital specialties), the properties of the PHQ-9 for major depression were consistent across this range.[14] The PHQ-2 consists of only the first 2 items of the PHQ-9; a PHQ-2 score of 3 or more has a sensitivity of 0.83 and a specificity of 0.92 for major depression.[15] The increased specificity of the PHQ-2 may be better for screening larger populations. However, a comparison of these 2 instruments has not yet been conducted. In addition, the PHQ-9 may also be used to monitor treatment response.

Other scales The Beck Depression Inventory for Primary Care is a 7-item scale adapted from the 21-item Beck Depression Inventory (BDI). It has a 0.97 sensitivity and 0.99 specificity for a score of 4 or more but requires a license fee for use.[16] The World Health Organization Five is a 5-item scale that was found to be slightly more sensitive but less specific than the brief PHQ in a study of 400 primary care patients.[17] There are increasing numbers of studies of its use in different populations, and it is also freely available online in all languages. The Mental Health Inventory is a 5-item mental health tool that was used as a comparison for the validity of the PHQ, but it is not specific for depression.[11] Single-question screening methods have a low sensitivity of 0.32 but a high specificity of 0.97 and thus cannot be relied on as an effective screening tool.[18]

Comparisons of the various screening instruments have been conducted. In 38 studies involving 32,000 patients in primary care settings, depression instruments were found to be comparably effective (this included PHQ-9, BDI, and the Geriatric Depression Screen, among others) with a median likelihood ratio positive of 3.3 and were quick to use (administration times ranged from <2 to 6 minutes).[19,20]

Effectiveness of screening for depression

Data are conflicting as to whether general population– or primary care–based screening leads to improved patient outcomes. A systematic review of randomized trials of screening questionnaires administered by research assistants did not show any change in physician diagnoses or interventions; these studies used the BDI, General Health Questionnaire, and the Zung Self-Rating Depression Scale.[21] A more recent review for the US Preventive Services Task Force (USPSTF) found that there was only one fair-quality randomized controlled trial that directly assessed whether screening for depression among adults in primary care reduces morbidity or mortality and showed mixed results.[22,23] Based on data from four different trials, screening was thought to be effective when ancillary staff was involved in depression care and extra efforts were made to enroll patients in specialty mental health treatment.[22] A Cochrane review in 2005 concluded that screening and case-finding instruments, when administered without any additional care structure, had little impact on the overall recognition rates of depression, management of depression (or intervention with antidepressants), and outcomes from depression.[24] No evidence was found to address the harms of screening specifically. Potential harms include stigma and psychological effects of false-positive results of diagnoses and unnecessary treatment with and exposure to side effects of antidepressant medications. Some studies, but not all, showed concern for a possible increase in upper gastrointestinal bleeding in older adults when taking selective serotonin reuptake inhibitors (SSRIs) and nonsteroidal antiinflammatory medications together.[22] There is no definitive evidence that suicidal behavior increases with second-generation SSRIs, although there is evidence that there is increased risk under the age of 25 years and decreased risk over the age of 65 years.[22]

Screening for depression was found to be cost-effective only in settings of high prevalence of depression and high treatment and remission rates. Costs were high for annual screening but were lower for screening every 5 years and only truly cost-effective for one-time screening.[25] Pearls for depression screening are listed in **Box 2**.

ANXIETY DISORDERS
Burden of Disease

Anxiety disorders have a 12-month prevalence of 18% and a lifetime prevalence as high as 29% (see **Table 2**).[5,8] Morbidity includes a high degree of interference with life activities; increased number of physician visits, especially if there are somatic symptoms; and decreased functional status.[1]

Box 2
Screening for depression: pearls

1. There is reasonable evidence to support screening general primary care populations for depression.

2. Although there are many published screening tools for depression, the PHQ-9 and the PHQ-2 are good choices because of their good operating characteristics, free availability, and ease of use for patient self-administration.

3. A cutoff score of 10 or more for the PHQ-9 (sensitivity and specificity 0.88) and 3 or more for the PHQ-2 (sensitivity 0.83, specificity 0.92) is reasonable in the general population. The PHQ-2 may be favored if time of administration or length of a questionnaire is a concern.

4. Efficacy is likely increased with access to treatment, including collaborative care models where available.

5. Consider assessment for suicidality and bipolar disorder for confirmed diagnoses.

6. Consider comorbid assessment for anxiety disorders, either after diagnosis of depression or as part of the initial screening strategy.

7. Consider screening in selected populations, include those with cardiovascular disease such as poststroke and post–myocardial infarction, central nervous system disease, chronic pain, and cancer.

Screening Tools

Beck anxiety inventory

Selected tools and considerations are listed in **Table 4**. The Beck Anxiety Inventory (BAI) is a 21-item, patient-completed questionnaire, developed to discriminate anxiety disorders from depressive disorders in an outpatient psychiatric clinic.[26] Its questions primarily report somatic symptoms. An abbreviated version, the Beck Anxiety Inventory-Primary Care (BAI-PC), has subsequently been developed, and, although

---

Table 4
Selected tools and considerations for screening for anxiety disorders

Population	Tools	Description
General population/ primary care	GAD-7 GAD-2	GAD-7 and GAD-2 freely available
Medical comorbidities	GAD-7, others	Consider assessment for chronic somatic symptoms such as headache syndromes, chronic pain, gastrointestinal disorders Somatic symptoms such as gastrointestinal symptoms have been found to have a high prevalence of anxiety disorders in primary care[78,79]
Addiction	GAD-7, GAD-2	Perform better as general screens for anxiety disorders than for GAD specifically[80]
Elderly	GAD-7 Geriatric Anxiety Inventory Short Form (GAI-SF)	Consider using a lower cutoff score of 5–7 if using the GAD-7 GAI-SF: sensitivity 0.75, specificity 0.84
Psychiatric comorbidities	GAD-7, others	Consider screening for those with depressive disorders, other anxiety spectrum disorders, PTSD

a follow-up study has been completed, it has not been extensively retested using diagnostic interviews as the gold standard.[27,28]

Hospital anxiety and depression scale
Hospital anxiety and depression scale (HADS) was developed to screen medical patients for psychiatric conditions. Despite its name, it has also been validated in primary care populations. The optimal cutoff score for the anxiety subscale (HADS-A) is approximately 8, with a sensitivity and specificity in the 0.70 to 0.90 range.[29]

Generalized anxiety disorder-7
GAD-7 is another patient-completed questionnaire (**Box 3**).[30] Unlike the BAI, its criteria closely mirror the DSM-IV definition of generalized anxiety disorder, with the exception that it asks for a symptom report for the prior 2 weeks rather than for 6 months. As would be expected, using higher cutoffs of the GAD-7 yields lower sensitivity but higher specificity. A follow-up study found that it also performed well in identifying PTSD, panic disorder, and social anxiety disorder, with a sensitivity of 0.80 and a specificity of 0.76 at a cutoff of 7; for GAD alone, a cutoff score of 10 maintained sensitivity while improving specificity.[1] This tool has been shortened further to the GAD-2, a 2-item questionnaire for which a score of 3 has a sensitivity of 0.86 and a specificity of 0.83 for generalized anxiety disorder.[1]

Multistage screening tools
The Symptom Driven Diagnostic System–Primary Care (SDDS-PC) was developed as a 16-item, patient-completed screening tool for multiple mental health disorders in primary care.[31] In the initial study, it had 0.85 sensitivity and 0.60 specificity for generalized anxiety disorder, with lower sensitivity and higher specificity for panic disorder.[31] Although the performance of SDDS-PC is comparable with that of GAD-7 as an initial screen, it was designed to necessitate nurse or physician follow-up using a proprietary assessment module. Similarly, the PRIME-MD tool, as discussed earlier for

---

Box 3
Generalized anxiety disorder-7

Over the Last 2 wk, How Often Have You Been Bothered by the Following Problems?	Not At All	Several Days	More Than Half the Days	Nearly Every Day
1. Feeling nervous, anxious or on edge	0	1	2	3
2. Not being able to stop or control worrying	0	1	2	3
3. Worrying too much about different things	0	1	2	3
4. Trouble relaxing	0	1	2	3
5. Being so restless that it is hard to sit still	0	1	2	3
6. Becoming easily annoyed or irritable	0	1	2	3
7. Feeling afraid as if something awful might happen	0	1	2	3
	0 +	____ +	____ +	____
				=Total Score: ____

If you checked off any problems, how difficult have these problems made it for you to do your work, take care of things at home, or get along with other people?

Not difficult at all   Somewhat difficult   Very difficult   Extremely difficult

From The Patient Health Questionnaire (PHQ) Screeners. Available at: http://www.phqscreeners.com/overview.aspx?Screener=03_GAD-7.

depression, also contains a screen for anxiety disorders but was designed to be used with additional modules.[9] The PRIME-MD later evolved into the PHQ and then the shorter PHQ-9 and GAD-7. Neither SDDS-PC nor PRIME-MD is freely available for routine use, and the efficacy of using only the screening portion of such tools for anxiety disorders in a real-world setting is unknown.

Effectiveness of Screening for Anxiety

There are few cost-benefit studies available to guide implementation of screening of anxiety and depression. Small ambulatory studies showed that screening for anxiety is feasible and led to increased diagnoses even in training clinics but lacked cost-effectiveness data.[32] The collaborative care model is likely an effective intervention for both depression and anxiety,[33] with data supporting cost-effectiveness for depression,[34] equivocal results for panic disorder,[35] but lacking adequate studies for other anxiety disorders. Cost-effectiveness data are needed, as screening may identify illness of lesser severity, whereas more severe illnesses may present clinically without the need for screening. The shorter screening tests such as the PHQ-9 and GAD-7 only take minutes for the patient to complete and the provider to review, and its perceived utility is acceptable to patients.[10] Pearls for anxiety disorder screening are shown in **Box 4**.

OTHER COMMON PSYCHIATRIC CONDITIONS

Common mental health conditions encountered in the primary care office setting, including the neurodevelopmental disorder adult attention-deficit and hyperactivity disorder (ADHD) and the trauma-related disorder PTSD, are briefly discussed in the following sections. Substance use disorder (formerly substance use and dependence in DMS-IV) is not covered in this review.

ADHD
Burden of Disease

ADHD was originally thought to be primarily a pediatric disorder, whereas 40% to 60% of children with ADHD have symptoms that persist into adulthood.[36,37] ADHD is thought to have a prevalence of approximately 4% in the adult population (see **Table 2**).[5] In adulthood, symptoms of hyperactivity are less pronounced compared

---

Box 4
Screening for anxiety disorders: pearls

1. Anxiety disorders are widely prevalent, and there are freely available screening tools for use in primary care settings.

2. Despite wide prevalence and availability of proven screening tools, there is no conclusive evidence to support cost-effectiveness of screening general populations for anxiety disorders.

3. The GAD-7, using a cutoff of 10 or more, is a reasonable screen for generalized anxiety disorder (sensitivity 0.89, specificity 0.82). If a shorter screen is desired, the 2-item GAD-2 at a cutoff of 3 or more is an option (sensitivity 0.86, specificity 0.83).

4. The GAD-7 also screens for other disorders, including panic disorder and PTSD; it is critical to follow up this screening tool with an accurate clinical assessment.

5. Although not specifically screening, consider assessment for anxiety disorders in patients presenting with unexplained somatic symptoms.

6. Consider screening in patients with other psychiatric conditions, including depression and PTSD, as well as substance use disorders.

with those of inattention.[37] The DSM-V diagnosis of ADHD emphasizes pervasive symptoms of inattention, hyperactivity, and impulsivity affecting least 2 domains of daily life (eg, work and home).[6] Diagnosis is based on clinical evaluation, which should include assessment of other psychiatric illnesses and substance abuse, impact of these symptoms on daily functioning, and a developmental history.

Screening Tools

Several self-reporting measures exist for ADHD, but none are sufficient for diagnosis alone. The New York University ADHD Program advocates the use of Adult Self-Report Scale V1.1 from WHO. It consists of a total of 18 questions that correlate to DSM diagnostic criteria for ADHD, and the screener portion has 6 questions that patients can self-report. In a small study of 154 respondents, the screener questions were found to have a sensitivity of 0.69 and a specificity of 1.0, with an accuracy of 98%.[38] Subsequent validity studies showed strong concordance with clinician diagnoses.[39,40]

The Wender Utah Rating Scale (WURS) was originally found to have a sensitivity of 0.86, but subsequent studies showed a sensitivity of 0.72 and a specificity of 0.58, suggesting that it misclassifies about half of those without ADHD.[41,42] The Connors' Adult ADHD Rating Scales (CAARS) has separate scales for the patient and for completion by an observer such as a spouse, friend, or parent, so that physicians can gather corroborative data. Each scale has a screening, short, and long form. The Current Symptoms Scale asks about adult patients' behaviors in the last 6 months. It also has a separate scale for patients and for an observer. It is unclear whether any of these scales are superior.[43] In a 2011 systematic review that included 14 scales for ADHD, CAARS and WURS had the best psychometric properties. Firm conclusions were limited because of the poor quality of many of the studies identified.[44]

Effectiveness of screening for ADHD

More data are needed to clarify the value of screening for ADHD and the best tool for screening. Controversy exists about the diagnosis given that the symptoms of ADHD are challenging to differentiate from those of other psychiatric diagnoses or substance abuse. The Adult Self-Report Scale Screener shows considerable promise, and physicians should be alerted to its potential and for clinical signs of ADHD in their patients (**Box 5**).

POSTTRAUMATIC STRESS DISORDER
Burden of Disease

The overall lifetime prevalence of PTSD is approximately 7%,[8] higher in veterans[45] and other risk groups. PTSD is associated with functional impairment, increased mental health care utilization, and increased psychiatric comorbidities.[45]

Box 5
Screening for ADHD: pearls

1. ADHD is now considered a neurodevelopmental disorder in the DSM-V, with a prevalence of approximately 4% in adults.

2. There are several screening tools published for ADHD for patient or caregiver/observer report. The Adult Self-Report Scale V1.1 from the World Health Organization is freely available.

3. Although there are available tools for screening for ADHD, there is not sufficient evidence with regard to burden of illness or cost-effectiveness to support screening general populations.

Screening Tools

Screening tools for conditions such as generalized anxiety disorder may also be effective at screening for PTSD. For the office-based setting, if screening for anxiety disorders is performed, then use of the GAD-7 is a reasonable option. There are numerous screening tools for PTSD specifically, with validation in different populations, including at-risk groups such as veterans. The US Department of Veterans Affairs endorses several screening tools, including the BAI-PC, PC-PTSD, Short Form of the PTSD Checklist–Civilian Version (PCL-C), Short Screening Scale for Short Post-Traumatic Stress Disorder Rating Interview (PTSD), Startle, Physiological arousal, Anger, and Numbness (SPAN), Short Post-Traumatic Stress Disorder Rating Interview (SPRINT), and the Trauma Screening Questionnaire.[46] Of these, the 4-item PC-PTSD (**Box 6**) is available online through the US Department of Veterans Affairs Web site[47] and has been widely used in the veterans affairs (VA) system, whereas the other tools are either proprietary or require request from the researchers.

The PC-PTSD has been validated in the primary care setting at the VA with a sensitivity of 0.78 and specificity of 0.87 at a recommended cutoff of 3 (out of 4).[48] Alternatively, there are PTSD-specific screens that are available online that patients may complete on their own. The VA patient portal uses a version of the 17-item PCL specific for the veteran population.[49] Each question has a 5-point Likert scale ranging from not at all to extremely for possible PTSD symptoms. The recommended cutoff ranges from 30 to 50, depending on the population studied and the

---

Box 6
Primary care PTSD screen

Description

The PC-PTSD is a 4-item screen that was designed for use in primary care and other medical settings and is currently used to screen for PTSD in veterans at the VA. The screen includes an introductory sentence to cue respondents to traumatic events. The authors suggest that in most circumstances the results of the PC-PTSD should be considered "positive" if a patient answers "yes" to any 3 items. Those screening positive should then be assessed with a structured interview for PTSD. The screen does not include a list of potentially traumatic events.

Scale

Instructions:
In your life, have you ever had any experience that was so frightening, horrible, or upsetting that, in the past month, you:

1. Have had nightmares about it or thought about it when you did not want to?
   YES/NO

2. Tried hard not to think about it or went out of your way to avoid situations that reminded you of it?
   YES/NO

3. Were constantly on guard, watchful, or easily startled?
   YES/NO

4. Felt numb or detached from others, activities, or your surroundings?
   YES/NO

Current research suggests that the results of the PC-PTSD should be considered "positive" if a patient answers "yes" to any three items.

From Prins A, Ouimette P, Kimerling R, et al. The primary care PTSD screen (PC–PTSD): development and operating characteristics. Prim Care Psych 2004;9(1):9–14.

gold standard used to evaluate it, although a repeat study found that a cutoff of 60 maximized diagnostic efficiency (percentage of cases correctly diagnosed), albeit at a low sensitivity of 0.56 and a specificity of 0.92.[50] For screening purposes, if identifying the greatest percentage of cases is prioritized, a lower cutoff may be considered.

Effectiveness of screening for PTSD
Use of PTSD screens in general primary care populations outside the VA setting is less certain. Unlike the VA system, many primary care systems may not have access to specialized PTSD treatment; screening may not be desired if there is not readily available and effective treatment. These tools (PC-PTSD, PCL) may be considered if the clinical presentation includes symptoms suggestive of PTSD, although such use would not be strictly screening. Although some online Web sites use the 17-item questionnaire, the 4-item PC-PTSD may be a better initial screen for an in-office setting, especially if it would take additional time to complete in conjunction with screens for other conditions (**Box 7**).

LIMITATIONS OF EXISTING EVIDENCE

Despite the burden of disease and the availability of effective screening tools, there are still significant considerations in implementing these tools in clinical practice.

Optimal Cutoffs for Screening Tools
Most questionnaire-based screening tools use a quantitative scoring system. Operating characteristics such as the area under the curve vary depending on the population studied and the gold standard used and accordingly affect the optimal cutoff score. In addition, there is a value judgment in defining the optimal cutoff score. If one places a priority on sensitivity, assuming there is a readily available way to identify true diagnoses, then one would seek a sensitivity more than 0.9 and accept a lower specificity; the positive likelihood ratio of a positive result at such a cutoff would generally be low. Conversely, one may attempt to optimize both the sensitivity and specificity, accepting a lower sensitivity to preserve a higher specificity. Using the GAD-7 as an example, a cutoff score of 5 for screening of generalized anxiety disorder alone yields a sensitivity of 0.97 and a specificity of 0.57, whereas the suggested cutoff score of 10 still preserves reasonable sensitivity of 0.89 but improves the specificity markedly to 0.82. Thus, it is straightforward to recommend a cutoff score of 10; the small decrement in sensitivity, still at nearly 0.90, is an acceptable trade-off to improve the specificity to more than 0.80. However, if one uses the GAD-7 as a combined screen for generalized anxiety disorder, panic disorder, social anxiety disorder, and

---

Box 7
Screening for PTSD: pearls

1. PTSD has a significant burden and there are freely available screening tools.

2. Despite its prevalence, the best evidence for testing and most common strategies use a targeted screening approach.

3. Screening is likely most effective when performed where there are adequate resources for treatment of PTSD.

4. The PC-PTSD is a short, 4-item, freely available screening tool that has a sensitivity of 0.78 and specificity of 0.87 at a recommended cutoff of 3/4, best studied in veterans.

PTSD, the choice of cutoff is a bit more difficult; the cutoff score of 5 has a 0.90 sensitivity and 0.63 specificity, but increasing the cutoff score to 10 markedly diminished the sensitivity to 0.68 while increasing the specificity to 0.88. Thus, if one uses the GAD-7 as a screen for these multiple anxiety spectrum conditions, a midrange cutoff of 7 (sensitivity 0.80, specificity 0.76) might be more reasonable. The cutoff score to be used depends on the intended clinical use.

Funding Source

Many screening tool studies, including the PRIME-MD (and subsequently the PHQ), GAD-7, SDDS-PC, and PDI-4, were developed in conjunction with pharmaceutical companies or had researchers with pharmaceutical company relationships, raising the possibility of bias toward increased diagnoses that would lead to increased drug therapy.

Screening for One Diagnosis or More

There remains a question as to whether screening tools are more useful to assess for a single diagnosis or whether it is better to screen for multiple diagnoses at once. Even screens for one type of disorder have been found to be effective as screens for other diagnoses, thus rendering a decreased specificity. The BAI, for example, was designed to distinguish between depression and anxiety but in other studies tested positive for both; similarly, a depression scale, the Center for Epidemiologic Studies Depression Scale (CES-D), tested positive for patients with anxiety.[51] The GAD-7 was developed to screen for generalized anxiety disorder, but it also could be used to simultaneously screen for panic disorder, social anxiety disorder, and PTSD. In addition to the effect screening multiple diagnoses might have on operating characteristics, one must also consider the time it takes to complete the screening tools, as well as the clinical capabilities to treat all the diagnoses effectively. Broader screens such as the PDI-4, a self-completed 17-item screening tool that screens for major depressive episode, generalized anxiety disorder, ADHD, and bipolar affective disorder type 1, and the My Mood Monitor checklist, which screens for depression, bipolar spectrum disorders, and anxiety disorders, may prove useful pending further validation studies.[52,53]

THE ELDERLY

Late-life depression is often underdiagnosed and subsequently undertreated. Well-studied tools in the geriatric population include the PHQ-9 and the 15-item Geriatric Depression Scale (GDS). In a study of persons 60 years or older from primary care practices, scores of greater than 5 on the GDS had a sensitivity of 0.92 and a specificity of 0.81 for major depression.[54] In elderly primary care patients, the PHQ-9 performed comparably to the PHQ-2 and the GDS for detecting major depression. The PHQ-9 performed comparably regardless of gender or race and was somewhat better for younger elders and for those with fewer chronic illnesses.[55] The PHQ-2 was also validated in 8000 adults older than 65 years.[56] Overall, any of these scales perform well for screening for depression in the elderly (**Table 3**).

Studies of anxiety screening tools tended to have younger patients, however, and there is some evidence that geriatric populations may require different screening cutoffs or instruments. In the elderly, anxiety disorders may have overlapping symptoms of chronic medical conditions, and cognitive impairment may further complicate accurate identification. In elderly patients, for example, the GAD-7 may require a lower cutoff of 5 to improve sensitivity while maintaining specificity.[57] Alternatively, other assessment tools such as the Geriatric Anxiety Inventory (GAI) and its 5-item short-ened version (GAI-SF) have been validated against DSM-IV diagnostic interviews with a sensitivity of 0.75 and specificity of 0.84 (see **Table 4**).[58,59]

TARGETED VERSUS GENERAL SCREENING

Should these screening tools be used for the general population, for targeted high-risk groups, or both? Depression and anxiety disorders are of sufficient prevalence that general primary care screening would seem reasonable, despite concerns of uncertainty regarding definitive cost-benefit results. Comorbid psychiatric illness is common both concurrently as well as associated with increased likelihood of another disorder arising later in life.[60,61] Thus, there is a rationale either to screen the general population for both depressive disorders and anxiety spectrum disorders simultaneously or to screen for the other if one disorder is diagnosed.

Medical conditions have been associated with both depression and anxiety. Certain populations have demonstrated high rates of depression in association with medical comorbidities such as cardiovascular diseases or common social risk factors such as in veterans (see **Table 3**). Anxiety disorders may have higher prevalence in patients with other medical or psychiatric diagnoses, and there is evidence of efficacy of screening in these populations (see **Table 4**). For anxiety disorders especially, testing in these populations is more problematic with regard to screening, as the somatic symptoms may be one of the primary manifestations of an underlying anxiety or depression spectrum disorder rather than a comorbidity—whether to call this screening may be merely semantic.

Finally, in the current Internet age, patients may complete screening tests online by their own initiative or prompted by insurance companies or employers and bring the results to the practitioner to review. In such settings, however, providers should clarify whether the patient completed the tool as a screen or because of a concern regarding symptoms.

NOVEL AND ALTERNATIVE SCREENING MODALITIES

In addition to traditional screening with fixed-length questionnaires given in an office-based setting, there has been development of newer techniques (**Table 5**), including computerized, adaptive testing using proprietary algorithms, screening outside of the clinic using screening tools on the Internet, or by telephone interview. Although promising, these methodologies continue to require further study and refinement.

RECOMMENDATIONS
General Recommendations

It is essential that a screening tool be recognized as just that, a screening process for which a positive test is not synonymous with a diagnosis but which requires additional evaluation by a trained clinician (**Box 8**). Although there are no precise data to clarify the optimal time to administer these screening tests, or in whom, preventative health visits provide an opportune time to administer screening in the general population, with consideration of targeted screening as other diagnoses arise. In most cases, these tests may be self-administered. Office staff may give these screening tools to patients with the intention to complete the test while in an appointment. Some of the screening tools have translations in multiple languages. These tests could be administered as part of a more comprehensive questionnaire that includes

Table 5
Newer methods for screening of common psychiatric conditions

Tool	Description	Potential Uses	Limitations
Computerized adaptive testing	Computer-based questions ask follow-up questions depending on the response. Duration may vary depending on assessed accuracy of diagnosis	Internet-based screening in the office or at home	Need for computer, language capabilities, not widely available
Telephone	Using same screening tools, but administered by phone	Outreach to patients with barriers to coming in to the office	Patients would still need to be seen to clarify diagnosis and to start treatment; uncertain utilization of recourses
Internet-based screening	Could be done by clinic, by Internet at large (eg, advocacy or nonprofit sites, but could also be from pharmaceutical companies), or by insurance companies	Patient completed, may be more efficient for patient to complete at home	Less data for real-world use and how to integrate into clinical setting

nonpsychiatric conditions, although it is uncertain whether that strategy will affect accuracy or completion rates of the psychiatric screening tool.

Depression Screening

Given inconclusive data on efficacy and cost-effectiveness, official recommendations for screening for depression differ widely. Data suggest that screening is most effective in a collaborative care model (ie, integrated care with a medical doctor, case manager, and mental health specialist).[33] Although the effectiveness of

Box 8
Screening for psychiatric conditions: general pearls

1. Published properties (sensitivity, specificity) of screening tools depend on the population studied and may be different in clinical practice.

2. Positive test results are not synonymous with a diagnosis. Positive screen results must be followed by clinical assessment for a diagnosis, as only a portion of patients testing positive have a confirmed diagnosis.

3. Increasingly, these tools are able to be self-administered by patients, either in a clinical encounter or outside the office.

4. As many of these tools are widely available on the Internet, patients may find these tools themselves and bring results to the attention of their providers.

5. The optimal time for and method of screening is unknown. Preventive health visits represent an opportunity to administer screening tests.

6. Consider targeted screening depending on the condition and the populations represented in a given clinical practice.

screening without ancillary staff support is unclear, screening with the tools currently available requires little investment on the part of the practitioner and confers minimal immediate harm to patients themselves. Therefore, it is reasonable to screen for depression in the primary care setting, although it is best when ancillary support staff and specialist referral are available. The most readily usable screening tool is likely the PHQ-9 given its free availability, brief administration time, correlation with the DSM-IV criteria, and ability to track progress. Many current electronic systems, such as that in the Veterans Administration, use the PHQ-2 as a preliminary screen/clinical reminder, which, if positive, prompts the physician or care provider to complete a PHQ-9 or conduct a more thorough clinical interview. One may consider screening in populations such as veterans, those with postmyocardial infarction, poststroke, selected other medical conditions, and those with comorbid psychiatric illness (see **Table 3**). Positive diagnoses on further assessment should be assessed for suicidality, and screening for bipolar disorder should also be considered (screening for bipolar disorder specifically is not reviewed in this article) (see **Box 2**).

Recommendations from major organizations
The USPSTF recommends routine depression screening for all average-risk patients when there is sufficient staff-assisted depression care supports in place to ensure proper diagnosis, treatment, and follow-up (**Table 6**).[62] In contrast, because of concerns for a high rate of false-positive diagnoses and harms of unnecessary treatment and absence of high-quality evidence for the effectiveness of screening for depression, the Canadian Task Force on Preventative Health Care (CTFPHC) revised its guidelines in 2013 and recommend against routine screening of average-risk and increased-risk individuals (although this is a weak recommendation based on very-low-quality evidence).[63] Neither the USPSTF nor the CTFPHC make any recommendations on which screening test to use. The United Kingdom National Institute for Health and Clinical Excellence (NICE) guidelines suggest a targeted approach, screening only those individuals at risk for depression (including those with a history of depression or a chronic physical health problem with functional impairment), using the 2 PHQ-2 questions for screening.[64]

Anxiety Screening
Although conclusive cost-effectiveness is lacking, given the prevalence of the disease, the available treatment, and the multitude of screening tools, it is reasonable to consider screening for anxiety disorders in the office-based setting. Owing to its ease of administration, good performance characteristics, and free distribution, the GAD-7 is a reasonable first screening tool for anxiety disorders in the primary care setting. In addition to considering use at preventive health visits, one may consider screening as an adjunctive tool in patients with depression, addiction, and unexplained somatic symptoms, with the caution that this strategy of use, while effective at identifying cases, is not well validated with respect to cost-effectiveness and patient outcomes. The ideal cutoff score for GAD-7 for generalized anxiety disorder is probably 10 or more, with a sensitivity of 0.89 and specificity of 0.82. If one's practice has sufficient resources to treat other anxiety spectrum disorders, it may be reasonable to use a lower cutoff point of 7 to provide more sensitivity in identifying the additional conditions of panic disorder, social anxiety disorder, and PTSD (0.80 sensitivity and 0.76 specificity). If screening a general population as part of other screening questions, the GAD-2 may be more feasible to administer in the office because of its shorter length, with a follow-up GAD-7 for positive screens.

Table 6

Recommendations from major organizations regarding screening for selected psychiatric conditions

Condition	Organization	Recommendation	Screening Tool	Strength of Recommendation
Depression	US Preventive Services Task Force (USPSTF) (2009)	Routine depression screening for all average-risk patients when there is sufficient staff-assisted depression care support in place to ensure proper diagnosis, treatment, and follow-up	Not specified	Grade B: Recommended, high certainty that the net benefit is moderate or moderate certainty that the net benefit is moderate to substantial
	Canadian Task Force on Preventative Health Care (CTFPHC) (2013)	Recommends against routine screening of average-risk and increased-risk individuals	N/A	Weak recommendation, very-low-quality evidence
	United Kingdom National Institute for Health and Clinical Excellence (NICE) (2009)	Screen those at risk for depression (ie, history of depression, diabetes or coronary heart disease, disability, or dementia)	PHQ-2	Not specified
Anxiety disorders	USPSTF	Not addressed	N/A	N/A
	CTFPHC	Not addressed	N/A	N/A
	United Kingdom National Institute for Health and Clinical Excellence (NICE) (2011)	Assess in "people presenting with anxiety or significant worry," in patients who seek care frequently who have somatic symptoms, chronic physical health problems, or "are repeatedly worrying about a wide range of different issues"[65]	None specified	Not specified

Recommendations from major organizations

The NICE guidelines from the United Kingdom recommend considering the diagnosis of GAD in "people presenting with anxiety or significant worry," and in patients who seek care frequently who have somatic symptoms, chronic physical health problems, or "are repeatedly worrying about a wide range of different issues" (see **Table 6**).[65] However, these guidelines do not advocate for a particular screening method. The USPSTF, in its recommendation for screening for depression, mentions anxiety as a comorbid psychological condition that may merit increased depression screening, but there is no separate screening guideline for anxiety disorders.[62] Guidelines will likely continue to evolve as more research into cost-effectiveness is conducted.

SUMMARY

Depression and anxiety disorders remain significant conditions in the primary care setting and in the general population. Screening tools for depression and anxiety disorders are freely available with acceptable sensitivity and specificity. Screening tools for other conditions including ADHD and PTSD also exist. Novel screening methods, including Internet-based and computerized adaptive testing, are in development and may be promising tools in the future. Despite the availability of these tools and a need to improve the mental health of patients, the utility of widespread use of screening for depression and anxiety disorders in the primary care, office-based setting is uncertain, and guidelines have reached different conclusions. The best evidence for cost-effectiveness currently is for screening of major depression as part of the collaborative care model for treatment. Targeted screening is another reasonable approach in patients with comorbid psychiatric conditions or certain medical conditions.

Despite unanswered questions, with further research, a growing literature, and increased awareness of mental health, there is every reason for optimism for the future of mental health screening.

REFERENCES

1. Kroenke K, Spitzer RL, Williams JB, et al. Anxiety disorders in primary care: prevalence, impairment, comorbidity, and detection. Ann Intern Med 2007;146(5):317–25.
2. González HM, Vega WA, Williams DR, et al. Depression care in the United States: too little for too few. Arch Gen Psychiatry 2010;67(1):37–46.
3. Dans LF, Silvestre MA, Dans AL. Trade-off between benefit and harm is crucial in health screening recommendations. Part I: general principles. J Clin Epidemiol 2011;64(3):231–9.
4. World Health Organization. The world health report 2001: mental health: new understanding, new hope. Geneva (Switzerland): 2001. p. 23–9.
5. Kessler RC, Chiu WT, Demler O, et al. Prevalence, severity, and comorbidity of 12-month DSM-IV disorders in the National Comorbidity Survey Replication. Arch Gen Psychiatry 2005;62:617–27.
6. First M, editor. American Psychiatric Association: diagnostic and statistical manual of mental disorders. 4th edition. 2000. Available at: http://STAT!Ref. On-line Electronic Medical Library.
7. American Psychiatry Association. Diagnostic and statistical manual of mental disorders. 4th Edition, Text Revision. Washington, DC, American Psychiatric Association, 2000. Available at: http://dsm.psychiatryonline.org/data/PDFS/dsm-iv_tr.pdf. Accessed June 25, 2014.

8. Kessler RC, Berglund P, Demler O, et al. Lifetime prevalence and age-of-onset distributions of DSM-IV disorders in the National Comorbidity Survey Replication. Arch Gen Psychiatry 2005;62(6):593–602.

9. Spitzer RL, Williams JB, Kroenke K, et al. Utility of a new procedure for diagnosing mental disorders in primary care. The PRIME-MD 1000 study. JAMA 1994;272(22):1749–56.

10. Spitzer RL, Kroenke K, Williams JB. Validation and utility of a self-report version of PRIME-MD: the PHQ primary care study. Primary Care Evaluation of Mental Disorders. Patient Health Questionnaire. JAMA 1999;282(18):1737–44.

11. Kroenke K, Spitzer RL, Williams JB. The PHQ-9. J Gen Intern Med 2001;16(9): 606–13.

12. Martin A, Rief W, Klaiberg A, et al. Validity of the brief patient health questionnaire mood scale (PHQ-9) in the general population. Gen Hosp Psychiatry 2006;28(1): 71–7.

13. Wittkampf KA, Naeije L, Schene AH, et al. Diagnostic accuracy of the mood module of the Patient Health Questionnaire: a systematic review. Gen Hosp Psychiatry 2007;29(5):388–95.

14. Gilbody S, Richards D, Brealey S, et al. Screening for depression in medical settings with the Patient Health Questionnaire (PHQ): a diagnostic meta-analysis. J Gen Intern Med 2007;22(11):1596–602.

15. Kroenke K, Spitzer RL, Williams JB. The patient health questionnaire-2: validity of a two-item depression screener. Med Care 2003;41(11):1284–92.

16. Steer RA, Cavalieri TA, Leonard DM, et al. Use of the beck depression inventory for primary care to screen for major depression disorders. Gen Hosp Psychiatry 1999;21(2):106–11.

17. Henkel V, Mergl R, Kohnen R, et al. Identifying depression in primary care: a comparison of different methods in a prospective cohort study. BMJ 2003;326(7382): 200–1.

18. Mitchell AJ, Coyne JC. Do ultra-short screening instruments accurately detect depression in primary care? A pooled analysis and meta-analysis of 22 studies. Br J Gen Pract 2007;57(535):144–51.

19. Williams JW, Pignone M, Ramirez G, et al. Identifying depression in primary care: a literature synthesis of case-finding instruments. Gen Hosp Psychiatry 2002; 24(4):225–37.

20. Williams JW, Noël PH, Cordes JA, et al. Is this patient clinically depressed? JAMA 2002;287(9):1160–70.

21. Gilbody SM, House AO, Sheldon TA. Routinely administered questionnaires for depression and anxiety: systematic review. BMJ 2001;322(7283):406–9.

22. O'Connor EA, Whitlock EP, Beil TL, et al. Screening for depression in adult patients in primary care settings: a systematic evidence review. Ann Intern Med 2009;151(11):793–803.

23. Williams JW, Mulrow CD, Kroenke K, et al. Case-finding for depression in primary care: a randomized trial. Am J Med 1999;106(1):36–43.

24. Gilbody S, House AO, Sheldon TA. Screening and case finding instruments for depression. Cochrane Database Syst Rev 2005;(4):CD002792.

25. Valenstein M, Vijan S, Zeber JE, et al. The cost-utility of screening for depression in primary care. Ann Intern Med 2001;134(5):345–60.

26. Beck AT, Epstein N, Brown G, et al. An inventory for measuring clinical anxiety: psychometric properties. J Consult Clin Psychol 1988;56(6):893–7.

27. Benjamin S, Herr NR, McDuffie J, et al. Performance characteristics of self-report instruments for diagnosing generalized anxiety and panic disorders in primary

care: a systematic review. Washington, DC: Department of Veterans Affairs (US); 2011.

28. Mori D, Lambert JF, Niles BL, et al. The BAI–PC as a screen for anxiety, depression, and PTSD in primary care - Springer. J Clin Psychol Med Settings 2003;10: 187–92.

29. Bjelland I, Dahl AA, Haug TT, et al. The validity of the Hospital Anxiety and Depression Scale. An updated literature review. J Psychosom Res 2002;52(2): 69–77.

30. Spitzer RL, Kroenke K, Williams JB, et al. A brief measure for assessing generalized anxiety disorder: the GAD-7. Arch Intern Med 2006;166(10):1092–7.

31. Broadhead WE, Leon AC, Weissman MM, et al. Development and validation of the SDDS-PC screen for multiple mental disorders in primary care. Arch Fam Med 1995;4(3):211–9.

32. Zupancic M, Yu S, Kandukuri R, et al. Practice-based learning and systems-based practice: detection and treatment monitoring of generalized anxiety and depression in primary care. J Grad Med Educ 2010;2(3):474–7.

33. Archer J, Bower P, Gilbody S, et al. Collaborative care for depression and anxiety problems. Cochrane Database Syst Rev 2012;(10):CD006525.

34. Katon WJ, Schoenbaum M, Fan MY, et al. Cost-effectiveness of improving primary care treatment of late-life depression. Arch Gen Psychiatry 2005;62(12):1313–20.

35. Katon WJ, Roy-Byrne P, Russo J, et al. Cost-effectiveness and cost offset of a collaborative care intervention for primary care patients with panic disorder. Arch Gen Psychiatry 2002;59(12):1098–104.

36. Faraone SV, Biederman J, Mick E. The age-dependent decline of attention-deficit hyperactivity disorder: a meta-analysis of follow-up studies. Psychol Med 2006; 36(2):159–65.

37. Solomon CG, Volkow ND, Swanson JM. Adult attention deficit–hyperactivity disorder. N Engl J Med 2013;369(20):1935–44.

38. Kessler RC, Adler L, AMES M, et al. The World Health Organization Adult ADHD Self-Report Scale (ASRS): a short screening scale for use in the general population. Psychol Med 1999;35(2):245–56.

39. Kessler RC, Adler LA, Gruber MJ, et al. Validity of the World Health Organization Adult ADHD Self-Report Scale (ASRS) Screener in a representative sample of health plan members. Int J Methods Psychiatr Res 2007;16(2):52–65.

40. Adler LA, Spencer T, Faraone SV, et al. Validity of pilot Adult ADHD Self-Report Scale (ASRS) to rate adult ADHD symptoms. Ann Clin Psychiatry 2006;18(3): 145–8.

41. Ward MF, Wender PH, Reimherr FW. The Wender Utah Rating Scale: an aid in the retrospective diagnosis of childhood attention-deficit hyperactivity disorder. Am J Psychiatry 1993;150(6):885–90.

42. McCann BS, Scheele L, Ward N, et al. Discriminant validity of the Wender Utah Rating Scale for attention-deficit/hyperactivity disorder in adults. J Neuropsychiatry Clin Neurosci 2000;12(2):240–5.

43. Murphy KR, Adler LA. Assessing attention-deficit/hyperactivity disorder in adults: focus on rating scales. J Clin Psychiatry 2004;65(Suppl 3):12–7.

44. Taylor A, Deb S, Unwin G. Scales for the identification of adults with attention-deficit hyperactivity disorder (ADHD): a systematic review. Res Dev Disabil 2011;32:924–38.

45. Magruder KM, Frueh BC, Knapp RG, et al. Prevalence of posttraumatic stress disorder in Veterans Affairs primary care clinics. Gen Hosp Psychiatry 2005; 27(3):169–79.

46. PTSD Screening Instruments - PTSD: National Center for PTSD [Internet]. Available at: http://www.ptsd.va.gov/professional/pages/assessments/list-screening-instruments.asp. Accessed January 12, 2014.

47. PTSD: National Center for PTSD [Internet]. Available at: http://www.ptsd.va.gov/professional/pages/assessments/pc-ptsd.asp. Accessed January 12, 2014.

48. Prins A, Ouimette P, Kimerling R, et al. The primary care PTSD screen (PC–PTSD): development and operating characteristics. Prim Care Psych 2004;9(1):9–14.

49. My HealtheVet [Internet]. Available at: https://www.myhealth.va.gov/mhv-portal-web/anonymous.portal?_nfpb=true&_pageLabel=mentalHealth&contentPage=mh_screening_tools/PTSD_SCREENING.HTML. Accessed January 12, 2014.

50. Keen SM, Kutter CJ, Niles BL, et al. Psychometric properties of PTSD Checklist in sample of male veterans. J Rehabil Res Dev 2008;45(3):465–74.

51. McQuaid JR, Stein MB, McCahill M, et al. Use of brief psychiatric screening measures in a primary care sample. Depress Anxiety 2000;12(1):21–9.

52. Houston JP, Kroenke K, Faries DE, et al. A provisional screening instrument for four common mental disorders in adult primary care patients. Psychosomatics 2011;52(1):48–55.

53. Gaynes BN, DeVeaugh-Geiss J, Weir S, et al. Feasibility and diagnostic validity of the M-3 checklist: a brief, self-rated screen for depressive, bipolar anxiety, and post-traumatic stress disorders in primary care. Ann Fam Med 2010;8(2): 160–9.

54. Lyness JM, Noel TK, Cox C, et al. Screening for depression in elderly primary care patients. A comparison of the Center for Epidemiologic Studies-Depression Scale and the Geriatric Depression Scale. Arch Intern Med 1997; 157(4):449–54.

55. Phelan E, Williams B, Meeker K, et al. A study of the diagnostic accuracy of the PHQ-9 in primary care elderly. BMC Fam Pract 2010;11(1):63.

56. Li C, Friedman B, Conwell Y, et al. Validity of the Patient Health Questionnaire 2 (PHQ-2) in Identifying Major Depression in Older People. J Am Geriatr Soc 2007;55(4):596–602.

57. Wild B, Eckl A, Herzog W, et al. Assessing generalized anxiety disorder in elderly people using the GAD-7 and GAD-2 scales: results of a validation study. Am J Geriatr Psychiatry 2013. [Epub ahead of print].

58. Pachana NA, Byrne GJ, Siddle H, et al. Development and validation of the Geriatric Anxiety Inventory. Int Psychogeriatr 2007;19(1):103–14.

59. Byrne GJ, Pachana NA. Development and validation of a short form of the Geriatric Anxiety Inventory–the GAI-SF. Int Psychogeriatr 2011;23(1):125–31.

60. Kessler RC, Berglund PA, Dewit DJ, et al. Distinguishing generalized anxiety disorder from major depression: prevalence and impairment from current pure and comorbid disorders in the US and Ontario. Int J Methods Psychiatr Res 2002; 11(3):99–111.

61. Kessler RC, Gruber M, Hettema JM, et al. Co-morbid major depression and generalized anxiety disorders in the National Comorbidity Survey follow-up. Psychol Med 2008;38(3):365–74.

62. U.S. Preventive Services Task Force. Screening for depression in adults: U.S. preventive services task force recommendation statement. Ann Intern Med 2009;151(11):784–92.

63. Canadian Task Force on Preventive Health Care, Joffres M, Jaramillo A, et al. Recommendations on screening for depression in adults. CMAJ 2013;185(9): 775–82.

64. National Institute for Health and Clinical Excellence. Depression: treatment and management of depression in adults and depression in adults with a chronic physical health problem. Manchester (United Kingdom): 2009. Available at: http://www.nice.org.uk/CG90. Accessed December 26, 2013.

65. National Collaborating Centre for Mental Health (UK). Generalised anxiety disorder in adults: management in primary, secondary and community care. National clinical guideline number 113. Leicester (United Kingdom): British Psychological Society & The Royal College of Psychiatrists; 2011.

66. Whooley MA, Avins AL, Miranda J, et al. Case-finding instruments for depression. Two questions are as good as many. J Gen Intern Med 1997;12(7):439–45.

67. VA/DoD essentials for depression screening and assessment in primary care. 2010. Available at: http://www.healthquality.va.gov/mdd/. Accessed December 26, 2013.

68. Moussavi S, Chatterji S, Verdes E, et al. Depression, chronic diseases, and decrements in health: results from the World Health Surveys. Lancet 2007;370(9590): 851–8.

69. Kravitz RL, Ford DE. Introduction: chronic medical conditions and depression—the view from primary care. Am J Med 2008;121(11):S1–7.

70. Katon WJ. Clinical and health services relationships between major depression, depressive symptoms, and general medical illness. Biol Psychiatry 2003;54(3):216–26.

71. Lichtman JH, Bigger JT, Blumenthal JA, et al. Depression and coronary heart disease: recommendations for screening, referral, and treatment: a science advisory from the American Heart Association Prevention Committee of the Council on Cardiovascular Nursing, Council on Clinical Cardiology, Council on Epidemiology and Prevention, and Interdisciplinary Council on Quality of Care and Outcomes Research: Endorsed by the American Psychiatric Association. Circulation 2008; 118(17):1768–75.

72. Hackett ML, Anderson CS, House A, et al. Interventions for treating depression after stroke. Cochrane Database Syst Rev 2008;(4):CD003437.

73. Glassman AH, O'Connor CM, Califf RM, et al. Sertraline treatment of major depression in patients with acute MI or unstable angina. JAMA 2002;288(6):701–9.

74. Ziegelstein RC. Depression in patients recovering from a myocardial infarction. JAMA 2001;286(13):1621–7.

75. Berkman LF, Blumenthal J, Burg M, et al. Effects of treating depression and low perceived social support on clinical events after myocardial infarction: the Enhancing Recovery in Coronary Heart Disease Patients (ENRICHD) Randomized Trial. JAMA 2003;289(23):3106–16.

76. Stafford L, Berk M, Jackson HJ. Validity of the Hospital Anxiety and Depression Scale and Patient Health Questionnaire-9 to screen for depression in patients with coronary artery disease. Gen Hosp Psychiatry 2007;29(5):417–24.

77. Kroenke K, Spitzer RL, Williams JB, et al. The patient health questionnaire somatic, anxiety, and depressive symptom scales: a systematic review. Gen Hosp Psychiatry 2010;32(4):345–59.

78. Löwe B, Spitzer RL, Williams JB, et al. Depression, anxiety and somatization in primary care: syndrome overlap and functional impairment. Gen Hosp Psychiatry 2008;30(3):191–9.

79. Mussell M, Kroenke K, Spitzer RL, et al. Gastrointestinal symptoms in primary care: prevalence and association with depression and anxiety. J Psychosom Res 2008;64(6):605–12.

80. Delgadillo J, Payne S, Gilbody S, et al. Brief case finding tools for anxiety disorders: validation of GAD-7 and GAD-2 in addictions treatment. Drug Alcohol Depend 2012;125:37–42.

Screening for Depression in the Primary Care Population

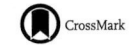

D. Edward Deneke, MD[a],*, Heather E. Schultz, MD, MPH[b],
Thomas E. Fluent, MD[a]

KEYWORDS

- Depression • Screening • Suicide • Primary care

KEY POINTS

- Depression is common in the primary care population, and imposes social, financial, and medical costs on patients on families.
- Screening for depression can be useful in the primary care setting if reliable systems of care are in place to ensure adequate treatment and follow-up.
- Use of collaborative care models for depression in the primary care setting have been shown to be a cost-effective means for providing depression-related care, but economic and cultural barriers continue to slow widespread adoption.
- Screening for suicide risk in the primary care population is generally not recommended. However, clinicians should familiarize themselves with the common risk factors for suicide and remain vigilant for patients at increased risk for self-harm.

INTRODUCTION

The *Diagnostic and Statistical Manual of Mental Disorders* (5th edition) defines major depressive disorder (MDD) as a mental health condition characterized by 5 or more of the following symptoms lasting for at least 2 weeks: depressed mood, diminished interest in activities (anhedonia), disordered sleep, fatigue, changes in appetite or changes in weight, persistent feelings of guilt or hopelessness, decreased concentration, psychomotor slowing, and thoughts of suicide; the 2 symptoms of depressed mood and anhedonia are cardinal, and at least 1 must be present for the diagnosis to be made (**Box 1**).[1] When assessing a patient for MDD, these symptoms need to

This article first appeared in Prim Care Clin Office Pract 2014;41(2):399–420.

Conflicts of Interest: None.

[a] Department of Psychiatry, University of Michigan Health System, University of Michigan, 4250 Plymouth Road, Ann Arbor, MI 48109-2700, USA; [b] Inpatient Psychiatry, University of Michigan Hospital and Health Systems, University of Michigan University Hospital, 9C 9150, 1500 East Medical Center Drive, SPC 5120, Ann Arbor MI 48109, USA

* Corresponding author.

E-mail address: edwardde@med.umich.edu

Psychiatr Clin N Am 38 (2015) 23–43

http://dx.doi.org/10.1016/j.psc.2014.11.006

0193-953X/15/$ – see front matter

Box 1
Diagnosing major depressive disorder

Five or more of the following symptoms are present during a 2-week period:

Note: Of the 5 symptoms, at least 1 must be depressed mood or anhedonia; symptoms need to represent a change from the patient's baseline, and be accompanied by an impairment in social or occupational functioning.

- Feeling depressed, sad, or hopeless most of the time (depressed mood)
- Decreased interest in pleasurable activities (anhedonia)
- Change in appetite (increase or decrease) and/or 5% or more change in weight
- Sleeping more or less often than usual
- Frequent feelings of worthlessness or excessive/inappropriate guilt
- Frequent fatigue
- Physical restlessness (psychomotor agitation) or slowed movements (psychomotor retardation)
- Indecisiveness or decreased concentration
- Recurrent thoughts of death or thoughts of suicide

From American Psychiatric Association, American Psychiatric Association DSM-5 Task Force. Diagnostic and statistical manual of mental disorders: DSM-5. 5th edition. Washington, DC: American Psychiatric Association; 2013.

---

represent a change from the patient's baseline, and must be accompanied by impairment in social or occupational functioning.

Depressive disorders are highly prevalent in the general population and can be found across the age spectrum.[2] The estimated lifetime prevalence of MDD in the United States is approximately 13.2%,[3] with a 12-month prevalence of 6% to 7%.[2] Evidence suggests that upward of three-quarters of those who experience a major depressive episode will experience a subsequent episode,[4] with the mean number of episodes among adults with lifetime MDD being 4.7.[3] Approximately one-third of nonelderly patients[5] and two-thirds of elderly patients[6] are treated in the primary care setting.

Somatic symptoms (eg, headache, back pain, fatigue, and other physical complaints) are frequently found alongside symptoms of depression, often dominating the clinical picture and masking the underlying depressive disorder. This masking can sometimes make an accurate diagnosis more difficult. A 2005 literature review reported that approximately two-thirds of patients with depression present to primary care with primarily somatic complaints, and the presence of somatic complaints correlated with a decrease in the clinician's ability to recognize the depression.[7] Somatic symptoms comorbid with depression have been shown to be more prevalent in certain populations, including those who are pregnant, elderly, poor, incarcerated, and those suffering from other medical issues.[7]

Depression has a significant impact on the lives of the affected population. Given the symptoms of the disorder it should not be surprising that people suffering from depression often experience a decreased quality of life, as well as decreased productivity both at work and at home.[8,9] Depression can also have a negative impact on a person's self-reported global heath rating, whether taken alone or in combination with common chronic health conditions (**Table 1**).[10] In addition to depression's negative impact on health, people with depression have also been shown to have increased mortality rates.[11]

Table 1
Global mean health score by disease status

	Mean Health Score[a]	
Chronic Condition	Condition Alone	Condition Plus Depression
Baseline	90.6[b]	72.9[c]
Asthma	80.3	65.4
Angina	79.6	65.8
Arthritis	79.3	67.1
Diabetes	78.9	58.5
Two or more chronic conditions	71.8	56.1

[a] Derived from 16 self-reported health questions; scores range from 0 (worst health) to 100 (best health); sample includes more than 250,000 people representing 60 countries.
[b] Health score for those with neither depression nor a chronic health condition.
[c] Health score for those with depression alone (no chronic health condition).
Adapted from Moussavi S, Chatterji S, Verdes E, et al. Depression, chronic diseases, and decrements in health: results from the World Health Surveys. Lancet 2007;370:851–8.

Depression not only affects the person directly suffering from the disorder but also family members, employers, and others with whom the depressed person interacts. Spouses of people with depression have been shown to experience increased symptoms of depression and an increased emotional and financial burden.[12] Children of parents with depression have been shown to be at increased risk of mental illness,[13] and to demonstrate changes in health care use including decreased well-visit appointments, increased sick visits to primary care, and increased use of emergency, inpatient, and specialty care services.[14] The economic impact of depression on society is also significantly large, with estimates suggesting annual costs may exceed $80 billion in the United States alone.[15] Although lost productivity explains the bulk of this cost,[16,17] estimates suggest that roughly 30% can be attributed to direct medical expenditures.[15]

Multiple risk factors for depression have been demonstrated in the literature (**Box 2**). Gender is a major risk factor, with the lifetime prevalence of MDD about twice as high for women than for men.[5] Rates of depression have also been found to be higher in

Box 2
Risk factors for depression

1. Family history of depression
2. Female gender
3. Poor social supports
4. Substance abuse
5. Prior depressive episode
6. Childhood trauma
7. Childbirth
8. Dementia
9. Stressful life events
10. Low socioeconomic status
11. Significant medical burden
12. Certain personality traits, such as low self-esteem or excessive pessimism

people with other psychiatric disorders, such as anxiety or substance-use disorders, and in people with comorbid medical issues or a family history of depression. Lower socioeconomic status and unemployment also appear to be risk factors for depression.[5] The average age of onset for depressive disorders is the mid-20s to 30s, with overall risk decreasing in the following decades.[5] Depression is less common in the community-living geriatric population, but clinicians should keep in mind that those who are elderly may be exposed to various age-specific risk factors, including loss of independence and increased medical burden.[13]

Depression has been found to be more common among whites than blacks, although depression in black populations has been found to be more severe and linked with greater functional impairment.[18] Racially linked disparities in severity and impairment are attributable, in part, to differences in securing necessary care.[19] Research suggests that treatment preferences and illness beliefs do not fully account for race-based differences in obtaining appropriate mental health care[20]; access-related factors such as the affordability, availability, accessibility, and acceptability of mental health care likely play a significant role.[21]

Depression is also associated with a variety of medical issues, and the relationship is particularly strong in diseases of the central nervous system such as traumatic brain injury,[22] stroke,[23] and Parkinson disease.[24] Specific life experiences have also been identified as risk factors for depression, including childbirth,[25] childhood trauma,[26] and stressful life events.[27] Genetics seem to play a significant role in the pathophysiology of depression. The concordance rate for depression among monozygotic twins was found to be 37% in a large Swedish study involving more than 15,000 sets of twins.[28] Of note, this study also found a significant difference in the hereditability of depression between men (42%) and women (29%). As with most medical conditions, the precise role of genetics remains a mystery, with no single depression gene having been found; it is likely that the phenotype of depression is the product of a complex interplay between genetic vulnerability, conferred by small effects from a large number of genes, and environmental exposures.

CURRENT PRACTICE PATTERNS

The demand for depression-related care and the provision of that care in office-based settings in the United States is substantial; for example, the estimated number of visits for depression in office-based settings increased from 14.4 million in 1987 to 24.5 million in 2001.[29] Over this same period, the proportion of depression-related visits decreased for psychiatrists while it increased for primary care physicians: whereas psychiatrists accounted for 44% of visits in 1987 and 29% in 2001, primary care physicians accounted for 50% in 1987 and 64% in 2001.[29] Data from 1998 to 2007 suggest that the increase in outpatient treatment of depression has slowed, with the number of Americans receiving such care increasing from about 6.5 million in 1998 to 8.7 million in 2007.[30] These important data suggest that the growth in care grew more quickly for several groups that have been historically underserved, including blacks, Hispanics, and men.[30] Despite these improvements, evidence suggests that a substantial number of people in the United States remain untreated for their depression-related symptoms.[30]

Literature documenting screening rates for depression in primary care is not readily available; however, a 2009 review investigating the efficacy of depression screening among adults in primary care suggests that general mental health screening rates may be as high as 74%.[31] The specific disorders being screened were not delineated, but the investigators reasoned that screening programs for depression were likely among the most common, given the prevalence of depression within the primary care patient population. This review identified a large sample study investigating depression screening among outpatients within the Veterans Health Administration (VHA).[31] The study found that of the 85% of eligible patients screened, nearly 9% screened positive; among those screening positive, however, only 54% received follow-up evaluation, 24% of whom were subsequently diagnosed with a depressive disorder.[32]

While the rate of unidentified cases of depression presenting to United States primary care settings remains understudied, findings from the 2009 review suggest many adults with depression, perhaps as many as 40%, may not be properly identified by their primary care provider.[31] Researchers found that younger patients and those with less severe symptoms were among the most likely to be missed.[31] Another review identified somatization as one of the most important contributors to missing a diagnosis of depression in primary care.[33] This finding is particularly noteworthy, as up to two-thirds of depressed patients primarily present with somatic symptoms.[33] A review investigating the accuracy of depression diagnoses within primary care in North America, Europe, and Australia concluded that about half of the individuals with depression were not properly detected. Moreover, the investigators found that the risk of misidentification (false positives) was greater than the risk of missing cases, suggesting that primary care providers may need to exercise increased caution when making a definitive diagnosis in those screening positive.[34] One strategy that may help to improve depression screening and diagnosis is enhancing the structures and processes of care; that is, making the settings that carry out screening (and subsequent care) work better.

EVIDENCE FOR SCREENING

Evidence for the effectiveness of depression screening in the general population has been mixed. A 2005 review explored the utility of screening or case-finding instruments to improve the detection and management of depression in nonspecialist (ie, primary care) settings. Only minimal evidence linking routine administration of depression screening tools to rates of detection or treatment outcomes was found.[35] The investigators strongly discouraged the use of screening and case-finding instruments as stand-alone tools to identify those with depression. A subsequent meta-analysis revealed similar findings, concluding that screening settings themselves need to change to yield better results.[36] Of note, both reviews excluded studies involving enhanced systems of care, such as those that use care managers to support the primary care clinician in diagnosing and treating depression.

Two additional systematic reviews, completed in 2002 and 2009, reached similar conclusions[31,37]; however, when studies involving enhanced systems of care were included, investigators found that depression screening programs were effective in identifying and treating depression. Enhanced systems were those that included support staff, such as care managers, to augment the depression-related care provided by the clinician. Support staff assist clinicians with several functions, including patient education and follow-up, adjusting treatment plans, serving as a link between patients and the multiple components of the health care system (eg, mental health specialists and the primary care clinician), and (sometimes) proving limited mental health treatment. A meta-analysis investigating the efficacy of enhanced systems concluded that such models can effectively achieve improvements in depression outcomes in a wide range of settings.[38]

Although depression screening in usual care settings may not be cost-effective,[39] emerging evidence suggests that one-time screening for depression in settings with effective treatment programs (eg, enhanced settings with structured depression care) can make economic sense.[40] Structured collaborative care models (see later discussion) show promise in terms of both improving the quality of care and cost-effectiveness.[41,42]

SCREENING TOOLS FOR DEPRESSION

Several screening tools are available for use in the primary care setting. These tools vary in both their number and focus of questions. A meta-analysis comparing 19 screening tools with the number of questions varying from 1 to 30 found the median sensitivity and specificity to be 85% and 74%, respectively, with no significant difference found between measures.[43] In addition, brief screening tools have been shown to be as accurate as lengthier tools in detecting depression.[44] With many screening options and little evidence to differentiate the measures, primary care clinicians can easily become confused when trying to decide which tool to use with their patients. Decisions are likely often based on the availability of a given screening tool, as well as its ease of use for both patients and clinicians. To help minimize possible confusion, this article limits discussion to the following 6 commonly used tools: Patient Health Questionnaire–9 (PHQ-9), Patient Health Questionnaire–2 (PHQ-2), Beck Depression Inventory (BDI), Hospital Anxiety and Depression Scale (HADS), Geriatric Depression Scale (GDS), and Edinburgh Postnatal Depression Scale (EPDS) (**Table 2**).

Patient Health Questionnaire

The PHQ-9 (Appendix 1) is a popular choice for primary care clinicians, in part because of its brevity and ease of scoring. The PHQ-9 consists of 9 questions rating the severity of depressive symptoms over the past 2 weeks, with a tenth question used to assess impact of these symptoms on functioning. The first 9 questions are answered from 0 (not at all) to 3 (nearly every day). The sum of the first 9 questions gives the total score, with a total score of 10 marking the cutoff for likely depression. In addition to being a useful screening tool, the PHQ-9 has been demonstrated to be an effective tool in monitoring depression over time.[45] The PHQ-9 has been shown to be useful in a variety of populations, including blacks, non-Hispanic whites, Latinos, and Chinese Americans.[46] The PHQ-9 has also been validated in postpartum and geriatric populations.[47]

The PHQ-2 is a brief variant of the PHQ-9, often used as an initial screen for depression. The PHQ-2 consists of the following 2 questions, reflecting the 2 cardinal symptoms of an MDD (depressed mood and anhedonia):

- During the last 2 weeks, how often have you been bothered by feeling down, depressed, or hopeless?

Table 2
Screening tools for depression

Screening Tool	No. of Items	Cutoff Score for Depression	Free for Clinical Use?
Patient Health Questionnaire–9	9	10 out of 21 possible points	Yes
Patient Health Questionnaire–2	2	3 out of 6 possible points	Yes
Hospital Anxiety and Depression Scale	14	8 out of 21 possible points	Yes
Beck Depression Inventory II	21	20 out of 63 possible points	No
Edinburgh Postnatal Depression Scale	10	10 out of 30 possible points	Yes
Geriatric Depression Scale–15	15	6 out of possible 15 points	Yes

- During the last 2 weeks, how often have you often been bothered by having little interest or pleasure in doing things?

Each question is answered from 0 to 3, as in the PHQ-9, and the scores are added together for the total score. A total score greater than or equal to 3 is considered a positive screen. Using the cutoff score of 3, the PHQ-2 has been shown to have sensitivity of 83% and specificity of 92%.[47] Given the brevity of the screening tool, the PHQ-2 is a tempting choice for primary care clinicians struggling with a busy practice and ever-increasing screening recommendations. A common practice in primary care settings is to administer the PHQ-2 to patients and follow up with a more thorough PHQ-9 with those patients screening positive. Both screening tools are readily accessible for no fee from the manufacturer. Multiple translations are also available.

Beck Depression Inventory

The BDI-II is a 21-item self-report tool widely used in research for measuring the symptoms of depression. A shorter 7-item version designed for the primary care setting, the BDI for Primary Care (BDI-PC), is also available.[48] The BDI-II and BDI-PC are only available via license, thus limiting their use in the primary care setting.

Hospital Anxiety and Depression Scale

The HADS is a 14-item self-report scale, including two 7-item subscales for depression and anxiety, specifically designed for evaluation of psychiatric symptoms in patients with medical comorbidities.[49] The depression subscale focuses primarily on anhedonia and does not cover somatic symptoms. The HADS is copyrighted by the original authors and is available free of charge for clinical use.[50]

Geriatric Depression Scale

The GDS (Appendix 2) was specifically designed to screen for depression in the elderly population. Owing to the increased prevalence of medical comorbidities and somatic symptoms in this population, less focus is placed on somatic symptoms in comparison with other common screening tools. The tool comes in 3 versions consisting of 30, 15, or 5 simple yes/no questions. The 15-item version was found to have greater sensitivity and specificity than the 30-item scale.[51] The GDS is available free of charge from the designers, and is offered in multiple translations.

Edinburgh Postnatal Depression Scale

The EPDS has been well validated in pregnant and postpartum women.[52] The tool consists of 10 questions related to various symptoms of depression. The questions on the EPDS focus less on somatic symptoms (eg, weight change, sleep disturbances) and instead concentrate on depressed mood and anhedonia. Answers are graded in severity and scored on a range from 0 to 3. A total score of greater than 10 indicates possible depression. A study published in 2008 found the EPDS to have greater accuracy in depression screening among postpartum women when compared with the PHQ-9.[53] Like the PHQ-9 and GDS, the EPDS is available free for use from the publisher.

PROFESSIONAL GROUP RECOMMENDATIONS

Recommendations from the United States Preventive Services Task Force (USPSTF) and National Institute for Health and Care Excellence guidelines are summarized in **Table 3**.

Table 3
Professional group recommendations

US Preventive Services Task Force Guidelines[a]		National Institute for Health and Care Excellence Guidelines[b]
Screen adults for depression when staff-assisted depression care supports are in place to assure accurate diagnosis, effective treatment, and follow-up	Evidence Grade B[c]	Be alert to possible depression (particularly in people with a history of depression or a chronic physical health problem with associated functional impairment); for a person who may have depression, conduct a comprehensive assessment that does not rely simply on a symptom count
Do not routinely screen adults for depression when staff-assisted depression care supports are not in place. There may be considerations that support screening for depression in an individual patient	Evidence Grade C[d]	Routine depression screening is not recommended
Screen adolescents (12–18 y) for major depressive disorder when systems are in place to ensure accurate diagnosis, psychotherapy (cognitive-behavioral or interpersonal), and follow-up	Evidence Grade B[c]	—
Current evidence is insufficient to assess the balance of benefits and harms of screening of children (7–11 y)	Evidence Grade I[e]	—

[a] From the US Preventive Services Task Force (USPSTF).[54,55]
[b] From the National Institute for Health and Care Excellence Guidelines.[56]
[c] The USPSTF recommends the service. There is high certainty that the net benefit is moderate or there is moderate certainty that the net benefit is moderate to substantial.
[d] Clinicians may provide this service to selected patients depending on individual circumstances. However, for most individuals without signs or symptoms there is likely to be only a small benefit from this service.
[e] The USPSTF concludes that the current evidence is insufficient to assess the balance of benefits and harms of the service. Evidence is lacking, of poor quality, or conflicting, and the balance of benefits and harms cannot be determined.

United States Preventive Services Task Force

The most recent recommendations from the USPSTF suggest screening adults for depression in clinical settings with staff-assisted care supports in place to ensure accurate diagnosis, effective treatment, and follow-up.[54] The complexity of these staff-assisted care systems vary by site, but generally consist of either nurses or social workers providing assistance to the primary care clinician via care management, care coordination, or direct mental health treatment. The USPSTF review indicates that in primary care settings with such systems, treatment with antidepressants, psychotherapy, or a combination of both decreases comorbidity and improves outcomes in adults identified through screening; by contrast, screening in settings without these systems shows minimal benefit. The USPSTF reported good evidence supporting the efficacy of both antidepressants and psychotherapy in treating adult patients with MDD. Reported risks of antidepressant use include a possible increase in suicidality, especially among younger adults (age 18–29 years), and upper gastrointestinal bleeding. The risk of such bleeding may be most elevated for older adults using selective serotonin reuptake inhibitors (SSRIs). The USPSTF found no studies including adverse events associated with screening.

The USPSTF also recommends screening adolescents aged 12 to 18 years for depression in clinical practices having systems (or referral systems) in place to ensure accurate diagnosis, psychotherapy (cognitive-behavioral or interpersonal therapy), and follow-up[55]; evidence was judged insufficient to balance the benefits and harms of depression screening in children aged 7 to 11 years. Although the USPSTF notes that SSRIs have been found to be helpful in treating some children and adolescents with MDD, SSRIs are also associated with an increased risk for suicidality and should therefore be used only under close clinical supervision. A variety of psychotherapies have also been shown to be beneficial for adolescents (eg, cognitive-behavioral, interpersonal), and potential harms of such therapies are judged to be small.

National Institute for Health and Clinical Excellence

The National Institute for Health and Clinical Excellence guidelines encourage a case-finding approach with at-risk groups, including patients with a history of depression, those with significant physical illness (particularly if associated with functional impairment and disability), and individuals with other mental health concerns such as dementia.[56,57] Patients with coronary heart disease and diabetes have been prioritized for screening. The following list outlines conditions or circumstances whereby screening should be strongly considered:

- Parkinson disease
- Dementia
- The puerperium
- Alcohol and drug abuse
- Abuse victims
- Physical disease such as cancer, cardiovascular disease, or diabetes
- Chronic pain
- Stressful home environments
- Elderly and socially isolated
- Multiple unexplained symptoms

CHANGES IN HEALTH CARE

The current consensus regarding depression screening in the primary care setting includes screening only if staff-assisted support systems are in place to provide accurate diagnosis, deliver effective treatment, and ensure follow-up. Providing access to comprehensive systems is not a minor feat, as access to mental health professionals is a large barrier to treatment.[58] Primary care is frequently the de facto provider for patients with depression but, despite strong efforts, a large number of cases of depression are missed or inadequately treated.[59]

Collaborative Care

Over the past several decades efforts have been made to develop effective systems of mental health care within the primary care setting. The evidence supports the use of staff-assisted support systems,[38,60] but substantial variation exists among these programs. The term collaborative care is often used to describe such programs, consisting of a multidisciplinary team tasked with providing quality depression care in the primary care setting (**Box 3**). A recent Cochrane review analyzed data from 79 randomized controlled trials of various collaborative care models, and concluded that "[c]ollaborative care is associated with significant improvement in depression and anxiety outcomes compared with usual care, and represents a useful addition to clinical pathways for adult patients with depression and anxiety."[60] Most care models detailed

> **Box 3**
> **Key components of collaborative care**
>
> 1. A multidisciplinary, multiprofessional approach, to include primary care physician and at least 1 other health professional, such as a care manager (nurse or social worker) and possibly a psychiatrist or psychologist
>
> 2. A management plan structured to include guidelines or protocols for evidence-based information, and pharmacologic and nonpharmacologic interventions
>
> 3. Organized, scheduled patient follow-ups, in person or by telephone
>
> 4. Enhanced interprofessional communication, to include team meetings, feedback, and so forth
>
> *From* Gunn J, Diggens J, Hegarty K, et al. A systematic review of complex system interventions designed to increase recovery from depression in primary care. BMC Health Serv Res 2006;6:88.

in this review consisted of a primary care clinician, a care manager (often a nurse or social worker), and a mental health specialist (MHS), usually a psychiatrist or psychologist embedded within the primary care setting. The roles of the primary care clinician are to refer the patient to the collaborative care program (usually through the help of screening tools), prescribe antidepressant medications as indicated, and consult regularly with the other team members. The care manager follows a panel of patients with a diagnosis of depression, providing disease education and self-management tools, motivating the patients for follow-up, and tracking outcome measurements such as PHQ-9 scores. The MHS meets regularly with the care manager to review cases, provides medication recommendations back to the primary care clinician for patients discussed with the care manager, and provides direct consultation with patients on an as-needed basis. Treatments offered to patients, including medications and psychotherapy, varied among systems. In most models, the MHS serves primarily a consultative role. The regularly scheduled (usually weekly) supervision between the MHS and the care manager allows the MHS to influence the care of a larger number of patients than would be possible the MHS were simply seeing all patients on his or her own.

Despite the significant evidence supporting the effectiveness of collaborative care models, dissemination has been slow. This lackluster performance is likely due, in part, to inflexible clinical care models, increased upfront costs of the model, and difficulty in developing a sustainable model in the traditional fee-for-service environments (eg, the collaborative care model could increase some nonbillable services, such as supervision between the MHS and the care manager).[61,62] However, upcoming changes to the United States health care system present significant opportunities for advancement of the collaborative care model for depression care.

Affordable Care Act and Accountable Care Organizations

The passage of the Patient Protection and Affordable Care Act (ACA) in 2010 will likely affect the United States health care system for the foreseeable future, influencing depression care in several ways. For example, the ACA will expand the size of the insured population, thus increasing the number of patients seeking or needing care for depression from an already strained system. This influx of patients highlights the need for emphasis on population-based care models. Moreover, opportunities for alternative funding structures will likely arise through the formation of Accountable Care Organizations (ACOs).

ACOs consist of groups of coordinated health care providers tasked with providing medical care for a specific population, with reimbursements tied to cost savings and defined quality measures. Through utilization of ACOs established under the ACA, health systems have the option to participate in shared savings programs, allowing for funding of innovative models, such as collaborative care models, that struggle to thrive in traditional funding environments. As part of the shared savings programs, ACOs will be expected to meet specific quality measures established by Centers for Medicare and Medicaid Services. Among the 33 quality measures set for ACOs, one is intended for care of depression: screening for depression in all patients age 12 years and older and documentation of follow-up plans.[63]

Patient-Centered Medical Homes

The patient-centered medical home (PCMH) is a new model of primary care that emphasizes the delivery of comprehensive, accessible, and patient-centered care to patients within the primary care setting.[64] PCMHs focus on managing chronic diseases within the primary care setting, and coordination of care among providers is essential in achieving these goals. Given the high prevalence of depression within the primary care setting, depression care programs are a natural fit for PCMHs.[65] Specifically, collaborative care models share many common traits with PCMHs, including emphasizing multidisciplinary team-based approaches and effective communication between team members.[66] Successful implementations of collaborative care models with the PCMH can be found in the literature.[38,67–69]

Electronic Health Record

Electronic Health Records (EHRs) have the potential to significantly improve the quality of health care through ensuring accurate documentation of diagnosis and providing decision support for clinicians.[70,71] Use of EHRs in the primary care setting has been shown to benefit depression management; for example, EHRs can be used to trigger and help facilitate depression screening,[72,73] notify the primary care clinician of a depression diagnosis, and enable both accurate documentation and the provision of appropriate care.[74] However, EHRs frequently do not allow for the use of outcomes measures, such as tracking PHQ-9 scores over time, thus limiting their utility in assessing a given patient's progress in real time and on demand.[75] Of importance, the presence of EHRs in and of themselves does not guarantee improvement in depression care[76,77]: they need to be tailored to the particular demands (and resources) of a given setting, and structured to provide clinicians and patients with the information required to make informed decisions. As adoption of EHRs increase, studies will be needed to better understand their role in depression care programs and how they can best support collaborative models of care.

IMPLEMENTATION OF DEPRESSION CARE PROGRAMS

Implementation of depression programs, including screening, staff-assisted care support, and collaborative models of care, can be challenging. Recommendations from the literature are sparse, but consensus on key implementation strategies can be found.[62,78] For depression programs to be successful, buy-in from clinic leadership is essential; having a designated program champion to oversee the implementation is also valuable. In deciding the overall structure of the program, leaders, champions, clinicians, and other team members should not start from scratch, but instead rely on available evidence-based models on which to build their own program. A variety of models can be found in the literature.[38,60] Each clinical site is unique, and the chosen model should be used as a template to be molded to the site's particular needs. Barriers to changing clinical processes can emerge on multiple levels, from patients and providers to health systems and insurance providers. It is important that those involved in implementing a change process both acknowledge and seek to understand emergent barriers so that they can be dealt with appropriately.[62]

SPECIAL NOTE: SUICIDE SCREENING
What is Suicide?

When discussing suicide and self-injurious behaviors, consistent use of definitions is important for clear clinical communication as well as data collection and research. Suicide is defined as death caused by self-directed injurious behavior with intent to die. A suicide attempt is a nonfatal, self-directed, potentially injurious behavior with intent to die. Suicidal ideation involves thinking about, considering, or planning for suicide.[79]

By contrast, nonsuicidal self-injury (also known as deliberate self-harm) is the intentional, direct destruction of body tissue without conscious suicidal intent. The function of self-injury is complex. For instance, it is often associated with a need for relief/release of emotional pain, to provide a sense of control, to punish oneself, or to show distress to others.[80] Examples include cutting or hitting oneself, or ingesting toxic substances without the intent to die.

Epidemiology

Suicide was the 10th overall leading cause of death in the United States in 2010, with 38,364 total deaths.[81] Of note, in persons aged 25 to 34 years suicide was the second leading cause of death after unintentional injury. In 2010, suicide accounted for more than 1.4 million years of potential life lost before age 85 years.[82] Furthermore, for every person who dies by suicide, more than 30 others attempt suicide.[83] However, approximately two-thirds of suicides occur on the first attempt.[84] Men have a higher number of completed suicides (as they often use lethal means such as firearms), although women have a higher number of attempts.[85] Suicide is also closely related to psychiatric illness, and hopelessness and previous suicide attempts have been identified as strong prospective risk factors for suicide.[86] Although the prevalence of suicide is 0.01% in the general population, the risk increases 10-fold in depressed adults.[87] A summary of major risk and protective factors for suicide are shown in **Table 4**.

The Role of Primary Care Providers in Suicide Prevention

As per the 2012 National Strategy for Suicide Prevention, a report of the US Surgeon General, both primary care and emergency medicine providers are encouraged to screen for suicidality to improve the likelihood that the person will receive appropriate evaluation and treatment. These recommendations included screening, training to recognize risk, accurate diagnoses, implementation of trauma-informed policies and practices, easy access to mental health referrals, education of the warning signs of suicide risk, and continued care/improved aftercare.[83]

Of special importance, most individuals who complete suicide have presented to their primary care physician within a month of their death.[88] Furthermore, between 2% and 3% of primary care patients report suicidal ideation in the past month.[87] However, there are many ways to screen patients for suicidal ideation. For instance, the phrases in **Table 5** have been found to have different sensitivity, specificity, and positive predictive value for detecting patients with a plan to commit suicide.[87]

US Preventive Services Task Force

The USPSTF concluded in 2004 that the evidence is insufficient to recommend for or against routine screening by primary care clinicians to detect suicide risk in the general population. This situation was again reviewed in 2013, and the drafted

Table 4
Summary of major risk and protective factors for suicide

Risk Factors	Protective Factors
Male gender	Female gender (although females are more likely to attempt)
Previous attempt	Family/social support
Suicidal ideation	Hopeful
Mental illness	Access to mental health care
Caucasian	Prohibitive cultural or religious beliefs
Social isolation	Restricted access to lethal means
Recent loss (job, divorce)	
Alcohol/substance abuse	
Impulsivity	
Access to lethal means	
Hopelessness	
Family history of suicide	
History of childhood maltreatment	
Local epidemics of suicide	
Limited/no access to mental health care	
Physical illness/pain	

From Centers for Disease Control and Prevention. Suicide: risk and protective factors. Available at: http://www.cdc.gov/violenceprevention/suicide/riskprotectivefactors.html. Accessed December 27, 2013.

recommendations indicated that: "There is insufficient evidence to conclude that screening adolescents, adults, and older adults in primary care adequately identifies patients at risk for suicide who would not otherwise be identified based on an existing mental health disorder, emotional distress, or previous suicide attempt."[89]

Table 5
Sensitivity, specificity, and predictive value for detecting patients with a plan to commit suicide

Phrase	Example Screening Question (To Provide a Clinical Example Only)	Sensitivity (%)	Specificity (%)	Positive Predictive Value (%)
"Thoughts of death"	Since your last visit have you had thoughts of death? What seems to trigger these thoughts?	100	81	5.9
"Wishing you were dead"	Do you ever find yourself wishing you were dead? If yes, explain how often this occurs? What makes this better/worse?	92	93	14
"Feeling suicidal"	Are you feeling suicidal? If yes, how often are you thinking of suicide? Do you have a plan? Do you have access to firearms or other lethal means?	83	98	30

Adapted from Gaynes BN, West SL, Ford CA, et al. Screening for suicide risk in adults: a summary of the evidence for the U.S. Preventive Services Task Force. Ann Intern Med 2004;140:822–35.

Practically speaking, the cost to clinicians of screening for suicide relates to the additional clinical time such screening requires. Among the trials reporting on potential negative effects of screening for patients, none found serious adverse effects.[89] For high-risk patients with a history of suicidal ideation or attempt, it is important that they do not have lethal means to harm themselves, such as firearms, poisons, or materials that could be used for hanging or suffocation.[90] Any patient who endorses active suicidal ideation should be specifically asked about access to lethal means and if they have a plan to harm themselves. Suicidal ideation with a plan and lethal means constitutes a psychiatric emergency warranting acute evaluation in the emergency department (by a psychiatrist, whenever possible).

Recommendations of Other Groups

- The American Academy of Child and Adolescent Psychiatry: Clinicians should be aware of patients at high risk for suicide.[91]
- The American Academy of Pediatrics: Pediatricians should ask questions about mood disorders, sexual orientation, suicidal thoughts, and other risk factors associated with suicide during routine health care visits.[92]
- The American Medical Association: All adolescents should be asked annually about behaviors or emotions that indicate recurrent or severe depression or risk of suicide. Physicians should screen for depression or suicidal risk in those with risk factors such as family dysfunction, declining school grades, and history of abuse.[93]

Confidentiality and Patient Safety

Although there are few exceptions to maintaining confidentiality within the doctor-patient relationship, most states have "duty to warn" and "duty to protect" laws. These laws often address potential harm not only to others but also to self. Physicians should be mindful of their state laws regarding special circumstances when confidentiality may be breached, and to whom the information can be given. Clinicians can refer to the National Conference of State Legislators for more information regarding the laws in their state: http://www.ncsl.org/issues-research/health/mental-health-professionals-duty-to-warn.aspx.

Resources for Suicidal Patients

Primary care physicians should be aware of local resources, such as crisis centers and psychiatric emergency departments, to which a suicidal patient might be referred. Any patient who screens positive for active suicidal ideation with a plan and access to lethal means should be treated emergently. If a patient is not currently suicidal, but has a history of suicide attempts or suicidal ideation, it is important to provide the number for the national suicide prevention lifeline.

- National Suicide Prevention Lifeline: 1-800-273-TALK (8255). This confidential service is available 24 hours per day, 7 days per week to those who are in emotional distress or suicidal crisis.

SUMMARY

Depression is common in the primary care setting, and can significantly affect patients and families in several ways. Somatic symptoms frequently mask the underlying depression, leading to challenges in accurate diagnoses. Most depressed patients receive care solely in primary care, making this setting the optimal place for the use of targeted interventions. Screening for depression is the first step in treating depression, but is insufficient in providing quality care if subsequent support is not in place.

Several effective screening measures exist, many of which are widely available for clinical use. In addition to screening, systems should be in place to help ensure that the patients follow through with the treatment plan. Various models of care have been discussed in the literature, but further changes to current clinical culture and funding structures are needed before widespread adoption of these innovative systems can take place.

Thoughts of suicide are not uncommon in the depressed population. The current evidence is inadequate to describe risks/benefits of suicide screening in the asymptomatic adult population. However, primary care providers might identify patients with multiple risk factors or who are in high levels of emotional distress, and refer them for further mental health evaluation (acutely if suicide risk is deemed imminent). Most effective treatments of suicidal patients involve psychotherapy, and the primary care provider can provide support, referrals, and coordination of care. It remains important to recognize warning signs for suicide, such as a patient who talks about death or threatens self-harm.

REFERENCES

1. American Psychiatric Association, American Psychiatric Association DSM-5 Task Force. Diagnostic and statistical manual of mental disorders: DSM-5. 5th edition. Washington, DC: American Psychiatric Association; 2013.
2. Kessler RC, Chiu WT, Demler O, et al. Prevalence, severity, and comorbidity of 12-month DSM-IV disorders in the National Comorbidity Survey Replication. Arch Gen Psychiatry 2005;62:617–27.
3. Hasin DS, Goodwin RD, Stinson FS, et al. Epidemiology of major depressive disorder: results from the National Epidemiologic Survey on Alcoholism and Related Conditions. Arch Gen Psychiatry 2005;62:1097–106.
4. Kessler RC, Zhao S, Blazer DG, et al. Prevalence, correlates, and course of minor depression and major depression in the National Comorbidity Survey. J Affect Disord 1997;45:19–30.
5. Kessler RC, Berglund P, Demler O, et al. The epidemiology of major depressive disorder: results from the National Comorbidity Survey Replication (NCS-R). JAMA 2003;289:3095–105.
6. Harman JS, Veazie PJ, Lyness JM. Primary care physician office visits for depression by older Americans. J Gen Intern Med 2006;21:926–30.
7. Tylee A, Gandhi P. The importance of somatic symptoms in depression in primary care. Prim Care Companion J Clin Psychiatry 2005;7:167–76.
8. Daly EJ, Trivedi MH, Wisniewski SR, et al. Health-related quality of life in depression: a STAR*D report. Ann Clin Psychiatry 2010;22:43–55.
9. Simon GE. Social and economic burden of mood disorders. Biol Psychiatry 2003; 54:208–15.
10. Moussavi S, Chatterji S, Verdes E, et al. Depression, chronic diseases, and decrements in health: results from the World Health Surveys. Lancet 2007;370:851–8.
11. Cuijpers P, Smit F. Excess mortality in depression: a meta-analysis of community studies. J Affect Disord 2002;72:227–36.
12. Benazon NR, Coyne JC. Living with a depressed spouse. J Fam Psychol 2000; 14:71–9.
13. Olfson M, Marcus SC, Druss B, et al. Parental depression, child mental health problems, and health care utilization. Med Care 2003;41:716–21.
14. Sills MR, Shetterly S, Xu S, et al. Association between parental depression and children's health care use. Pediatrics 2007;119:e829–36.

15. Donohue JM, Pincus HA. Reducing the societal burden of depression: a review of economic costs, quality of care and effects of treatment. Pharmacoeconomics 2007;25:7–24.
16. Wang PS, Simon G, Kessler RC. The economic burden of depression and the cost-effectiveness of treatment. Int J Methods Psychiatr Res 2003;12:22–33.
17. Stewart WF, Ricci JA, Chee E, et al. Cost of lost productive work time among US workers with depression. JAMA 2003;289:3135–44.
18. Williams DR, Gonzalez HM, Neighbors H, et al. Prevalence and distribution of major depressive disorder in African Americans, Caribbean blacks, and non-Hispanic whites: results from the National Survey of American Life. Arch Gen Psychiatry 2007;64:305–15.
19. Miranda J, Cooper LA. Disparities in care for depression among primary care patients. J Gen Intern Med 2004;19:120–6.
20. Hunt J, Sullivan G, Chavira DA, et al. Race and beliefs about mental health treatment among anxious primary care patients. J Nerv Ment Dis 2013;201:188–95.
21. Cook BL, Doksum T, Chen CN, et al. The role of provider supply and organization in reducing racial/ethnic disparities in mental health care in the U.S. Soc Sci Med 2013;84:102–9.
22. Jorge RE, Robinson RG, Moser D, et al. Major depression following traumatic brain injury. Arch Gen Psychiatry 2004;61:42–50.
23. Robinson RG. Poststroke depression: prevalence, diagnosis, treatment, and disease progression. Biol Psychiatry 2003;54:376–87.
24. McDonald WM, Richard IH, DeLong MR. Prevalence, etiology, and treatment of depression in Parkinson's disease. Biol Psychiatry 2003;54:363–75.
25. Marcus SM, Flynn HA, Blow FC, et al. Depressive symptoms among pregnant women screened in obstetrics settings. J Womens Health (Larchmt) 2003;12:373–80.
26. Green JG, McLaughlin KA, Berglund PA, et al. Childhood adversities and adult psychiatric disorders in the national comorbidity survey replication I: associations with first onset of DSM-IV disorders. Arch Gen Psychiatry 2010;67:113–23.
27. Kendler KS, Karkowski LM, Prescott CA. Causal relationship between stressful life events and the onset of major depression. Am J Psychiatry 1999;156:837–41.
28. Kendler KS, Gatz M, Gardner CO, et al. Swedish national twin study of lifetime major depression. Am J Psychiatry 2006;163:109–14.
29. Stafford RS, MacDonald EA, Finkelstein SN. National patterns of medication treatment for depression, 1987 to 2001. Prim Care Companion J Clin Psychiatry 2001; 3:232–5.
30. Marcus SC, Olfson M. National trends in the treatment for depression from 1998 to 2007. Arch Gen Psychiatry 2010;67:1265–73.
31. O'Connor EA, Whitlock EP, Gaynes B, et al. Screening for depression in adults and older adults in primary care: an updated systematic review. Rockville (MD): 2009.
32. Desai MM, Rosenheck RA, Craig TJ. Case-finding for depression among medical outpatients in the Veterans Health Administration. Med Care 2006;44:175–81.
33. Timonen M, Liukkonen T. Management of depression in adults. BMJ 2008;336:435–9.
34. Mitchell AJ, Vaze A, Rao S. Clinical diagnosis of depression in primary care: a meta-analysis. Lancet 2009;374:609–19.
35. Gilbody S, House AO, Sheldon TA. Screening and case finding instruments for depression. Cochrane Database Syst Rev 2005;(4):CD002792.
36. Gilbody S, Sheldon T, House A. Screening and case-finding instruments for depression: a meta-analysis. CMAJ 2008;178:997–1003.
37. Pignone M, Gaynes BN, Rushton JL, et al. Screening for depression. Rockville (MD): 2002.

38. Thota AB, Sipe TA, Byard GJ, et al. Collaborative care to improve the management of depressive disorders: a community guide systematic review and meta-analysis. Am J Prev Med 2012;42:525–38.
39. Paulden M, Palmer S, Hewitt C, et al. Screening for postnatal depression in primary care: cost effectiveness analysis. BMJ 2009;339:b5203.
40. Valenstein M, Vijan S, Zeber JE, et al. The cost-utility of screening for depression in primary care. Ann Intern Med 2001;134:345–60.
41. Unutzer J, Katon WJ, Fan MY, et al. Long-term cost effects of collaborative care for late-life depression. Am J Manag Care 2008;14:95–100.
42. Katon W, Russo J, Lin EH, et al. Cost-effectiveness of a multicondition collaborative care intervention: a randomized controlled trial. Arch Gen Psychiatry 2012; 69:506–14.
43. Williams JW Jr, Pignone M, Ramirez G, et al. Identifying depression in primary care: a literature synthesis of case-finding instruments. Gen Hosp Psychiatry 2002;24:225–37.
44. Akena D, Joska J, Obuku EA, et al. Comparing the accuracy of brief versus long depression screening instruments which have been validated in low and middle income countries: a systematic review. BMC Psychiatry 2012;12:187.
45. Kroenke K, Spitzer RL, Williams JB, et al. The patient health questionnaire somatic, anxiety, and depressive symptom scales: a systematic review. Gen Hosp Psychiatry 2010;32:345–59.
46. Huang FY, Chung H, Kroenke K, et al. Using the Patient Health Questionnaire-9 to measure depression among racially and ethnically diverse primary care patients. J Gen Intern Med 2006;21:547–52.
47. Kroenke K, Spitzer RL, Williams JB. The Patient Health Questionnaire-2: validity of a two-item depression screener. Med Care 2003;41:1284–92.
48. Steer RA, Cavalieri TA, Leonard DM, et al. Use of the Beck Depression Inventory for Primary Care to screen for major depression disorders. Gen Hosp Psychiatry 1999;21:106–11.
49. Herrmann C. International experiences with the Hospital Anxiety and Depression Scale—a review of validation data and clinical results. J Psychosom Res 1997;42: 17–41.
50. Mapi Research Trust. HADS (Hospital Anxiety and Depression Scale). Available at: http://www.mapi-trust.org/services/questionnairelicensing/catalog-questionnaires/240-hads. Accessed October 25, 2013.
51. Mitchell AJ, Bird V, Rizzo M, et al. Diagnostic validity and added value of the Geriatric Depression Scale for depression in primary care: a meta-analysis of GDS30 and GDS15. J Affect Disord 2010;125:10–7.
52. Hewitt C, Gilbody S, Brealey S, et al. Methods to identify postnatal depression in primary care: an integrated evidence synthesis and value of information analysis. Health Technol Assess 2009;13:1–145, 147–230.
53. Hanusa BH, Scholle SH, Haskett RF, et al. Screening for depression in the postpartum period: a comparison of three instruments. J Womens Health (Larchmt) 2008;17:585–96.
54. U.S. Preventive Services Task Force. Screening for depression in adults: recommendation statement. 2009. Available at: http://www.uspreventiveservicestaskforce.org/uspstf09/adultdepression/addeprrs.htm. Accessed October 10, 2013.
55. U.S. Preventive Services Task Force. Screening and treatment for major depressive disorder in children and adolescents: recommendation statement. 2009. Available at: http://www.uspreventiveservicestaskforce.org/uspstf09/depression/chdeprrs.htm. Accessed October 10, 2013.

56. National Institute for Health and Clinical Excellence. Treatment and management of depression in adults, including adults with a chronic physical health problem. 2009. Available at: http://www.nice.org.uk/nicemedia/live/12329/45890/45890.pdf. Accessed December 27, 2013.

57. Pilling S, Anderson I, Goldberg D, et al. Depression in adults, including those with a chronic physical health problem: summary of NICE guidance. BMJ 2009;339:b4108.

58. Cunningham PJ. Beyond parity: primary care physicians' perspectives on access to mental health care. Health Aff (Millwood) 2009;28:w490–501.

59. Olfson M, Marcus SC, Tedeschi M, et al. Continuity of antidepressant treatment for adults with depression in the United States. Am J Psychiatry 2006;163:101–8.

60. Archer J, Bower P, Gilbody S, et al. Collaborative care for depression and anxiety problems. Cochrane Database Syst Rev 2012;(10):CD006525.

61. Bachman J, Pincus HA, Houtsinger JK, et al. Funding mechanisms for depression care management: opportunities and challenges. Gen Hosp Psychiatry 2006;28:278–88.

62. Pincus HA, Pechura CM, Elinson L, et al. Depression in primary care: linking clinical and systems strategies. Gen Hosp Psychiatry 2001;23:311–8.

63. RTI International, Telligen. Accountable Care Organization 2013 program analysis: quality performance standards narrative measure specifications. Research Triangle Park (NC): 2012.

64. Agency for Healthcare Research and Quality. Defining the PCMH. Available at: http://pcmh.ahrq.gov/page/defining-pcmh. Accessed December 8, 2013.

65. Croghan TW, Brown JD. Integrating mental health treatment into the patient centered medical home. Rockville (MD): Agency for Healthcare Research and Quality; 2010. AHRQ Publication No. 10-0084-EF.

66. Gunn J, Diggens J, Hegarty K, et al. A systematic review of complex system interventions designed to increase recovery from depression in primary care. BMC Health Serv Res 2006;6:88.

67. Baik SY, Crabtree BF, Gonzales JJ. Primary care clinicians' recognition and management of depression: a model of depression care in real-world primary care practice. J Gen Intern Med 2013;28:1430–9.

68. Crabtree BF, Nutting PA, Miller WL, et al. Summary of the National Demonstration Project and recommendations for the patient-centered medical home. Ann Fam Med 2010;8(Suppl 1):S80–90 S92.

69. Chung H, Kim A, Neighbors CJ, et al. Early experience of a pilot intervention for patients with depression and chronic medical illness in an urban ACO. Gen Hosp Psychiatry 2013;35:468–71.

70. Institute of Medicine. Crossing the quality chasm: a new health system for the 21st century. Washington, DC: 2001.

71. Blumenthal D, Tavenner M. The "meaningful use" regulation for electronic health records. N Engl J Med 2010;363:501–4.

72. Klein EW, Hunt JS, Leblanc BH. Depression screening interfaced with an electronic health record: a feasibility study in a primary care clinic using optical mark reader technology. Prim Care Companion J Clin Psychiatry 2006;8:324–8.

73. Gill JM, Dansky BS. Use of an electronic medical record to facilitate screening for depression in primary care. Prim Care Companion J Clin Psychiatry 2003;5:125–8.

74. Rollman BL, Hanusa BH, Gilbert T, et al. The electronic medical record. A randomized trial of its impact on primary care physicians' initial management of major depression [corrected]. Arch Intern Med 2001;161:189–97.

75. Kobus AM, Harman JS, Do HD, et al. Challenges to depression care documentation in an EHR. Fam Med 2013;45:268–71.

76. Harman JS, Rost KM, Harle CA, et al. Electronic medical record availability and primary care depression treatment. J Gen Intern Med 2012;27:962–7.
77. Rollman BL, Hanusa BH, Lowe HJ, et al. A randomized trial using computerized decision support to improve treatment of major depression in primary care. J Gen Intern Med 2002;17:493–503.
78. Rollman BL, Weinreb L, Korsen N, et al. Implementation of guideline-based care for depression in primary care. Adm Policy Ment Health 2006;33:43–53.
79. Centers for Disease Control and Prevention. Definitions: self-inflicted violence. 2012. Available at: http://www.cdc.gov/violenceprevention/suicide/definitions. html. Accessed October 10, 2013.
80. Lloyd-Richardson EE, Perrine N, Dierker L, et al. Characteristics and functions of non-suicidal self-injury in a community sample of adolescents. Psychol Med 2007;37:1183–92.
81. Centers for Disease Control and Prevention. 10 leading causes of death by age group—2010. Available at: http://www.cdc.gov/injury/wisqars/pdf/10LCID_All_Deaths_By_Age_Group_2010-a.pdf. Accessed October 10, 2013.
82. Centers for Disease Control and Prevention. Years of potential life lost (YLL) reports, 1999-2010. Available at: http://webappa.cdc.gov/sasweb/ncipc/ypll10. html. Accessed October 10, 2013.
83. U.S. Department of Health and Human Services (HHS) Office of the Surgeon General and National Action Alliance for Suicide Prevention. 2012 national strategy for suicide prevention: goals and objectives for action: a report of the U.S. Surgeon General and of the National Action Alliance for Suicide Prevention. Washington, DC: HHS; 2012.
84. Mann JJ. A current perspective of suicide and attempted suicide. Ann Intern Med 2002;136:302–11.
85. Nock MK, Borges G, Bromet EJ, et al. Suicide and suicidal behavior. Epidemiol Rev 2008;30:133–54.
86. Brown GK, Beck AT, Steer RA, et al. Risk factors for suicide in psychiatric outpatients: a 20-year prospective study. J Consult Clin Psychol 2000;68:371–7.
87. Gaynes BN, West SL, Ford CA, et al. Screening for suicide risk in adults: a summary of the evidence for the U.S. Preventive Services Task Force. Ann Intern Med 2004;140:822–35.
88. Luoma JB, Martin CE, Pearson JL. Contact with mental health and primary care providers before suicide: a review of the evidence. Am J Psychiatry 2002;159: 909–16.
89. U.S. Preventive Services Task Force. Screening for suicide risk in adolescents, adults, and older adults: draft recommendation statement. 2013. Available at: http://www. uspreventiveservicestaskforce.org/uspstf13/suicide/suicidedraftrec.htm. Accessed October 10, 2013.
90. Mann JJ, Apter A, Bertolote J, et al. Suicide prevention strategies: a systematic review. JAMA 2005;294:2064–74.
91. Suicide and suicide attempts in adolescents. Committee on Adolescents. American Academy of Pediatrics. Pediatrics 2000;105:871–4.
92. American Academy of Child and Adolescent Psychiatry. Practice parameter for the assessment and treatment of children and adolescents with suicidal behavior. American Academy of Child and Adolescent Psychiatry. J Am Acad Child Adolesc Psychiatry 2001;40:24S–51S.
93. American Medical Association, Department of Adolescent Health. Guidelines for adolescent preventive services (GAPS): recommendations monograph. 2nd edition. Chicago: American Medical Association, Dept. of Adolescent Health; 1995.

APPENDIX 1: PATIENT HEALTH QUESTIONNAIRE–9

PATIENT HEALTH QUESTIONNAIRE-9 (PHQ-9)

Over the <u>last 2 weeks</u>, how often have you been bothered by any of the following problems? *(Use "✔" to indicate your answer)*	Not at all	Several days	More than half the days	Nearly every day
1. Little interest or pleasure in doing things	0	1	2	3
2. Feeling down, depressed, or hopeless	0	1	2	3
3. Trouble falling or staying asleep, or sleeping too much	0	1	2	3
4. Feeling tired or having little energy	0	1	2	3
5. Poor appetite or overeating	0	1	2	3
6. Feeling bad about yourself — or that you are a failure or have let yourself or your family down	0	1	2	3
7. Trouble concentrating on things, such as reading the newspaper or watching television	0	1	2	3
8. Moving or speaking so slowly that other people could have noticed? Or the opposite — being so fidgety or restless that you have been moving around a lot more than usual	0	1	2	3
9. Thoughts that you would be better off dead or of hurting yourself in some way	0	1	2	3

FOR OFFICE CODING ___0___ + _____ + _____ + _____

=Total Score: _____

If you checked off <u>any</u> problems, how <u>difficult</u> have these problems made it for you to do your work, take care of things at home, or get along with other people?

Not difficult at all	Somewhat difficult	Very difficult	Extremely difficult
☐	☐	☐	☐

Developed by Drs. Robert L. Spitzer, Janet B.W. Williams, Kurt Kroenke and colleagues, with an educational grant from Pfizer Inc. No permission required to reproduce, translate, display or distribute.

From Patient Health Questionnaire Screeners. Available at: http://www.phqscreeners.com/overview.aspx?Screener=02_PHQ-9.

APPENDIX 2: GERIATRIC DEPRESSION SCALE, SHORT FORM
MOOD SCALE (short form)
Choose the best answer for how you have felt over the past week:
1. Are you basically satisfied with your life? YES/NO

2. Have you dropped many of your activities and interests? YES/NO
3. Do you feel that your life is empty? YES/NO
4. Do you often get bored? YES/NO
5. Are you in good spirits most of the time? YES/NO
6. Are you afraid that something bad is going to happen to you? YES/NO
7. Do you feel happy most of the time? YES/NO
8. Do you often feel helpless? YES/NO
9. Do you prefer to stay at home, rather than going out and doing new things? YES/NO
10. Do you feel you have more problems with memory than most? YES/NO
11. Do you think it is wonderful to be alive now? YES/NO
12. Do you feel pretty worthless the way you are now? YES/NO
13. Do you feel full of energy? YES/NO
14. Do you feel that your situation is hopeless? YES/NO
15. Do you think that most people are better off than you are? YES/NO

From Geriatric Depression Scale. Available at: http://www.stanford.edu/~yesavage/GDS.english.short.html.

Posttraumatic Stress in Older Adults

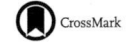

When Medical Diagnoses or Treatments Cause Traumatic Stress

Jennifer Moye, PhD[a,b,]*, Susan J. Rouse, PMH-CNS-BC[a]

KEYWORDS

- Posttraumatic stress disorder (PTSD) • Geriatric • Cardiac • Cancer

KEY POINTS

- Most older patients adapt after catastrophic medical diagnoses and treatments, but a significant number may develop posttraumatic stress disorder (PTSD) symptoms.
- PTSD symptoms create added burden for the individual, family, and health care system for the patient's recovery.
- Medical-related PTSD may be underdiagnosed by providers who may be unaware that these health problems can lead to PTSD symptoms.
- Treatment research is lacking, but pharmacologic and nonpharmacologic approaches to treatment may be extrapolated and adjusted from the literature focusing on younger adults.
- Additional study is needed.

INTRODUCTION
The Condition

The most familiar form of posttraumatic stress disorder (PTSD) occurs in veterans exposed to combat, and it can recur or worsen in the setting of other stressors in late life, including medical illness. This article draws attention to a different and under-appreciated problem of posttraumatic stress symptoms (PTSSs) and PTSD arising from catastrophic medical illness.

In the latest edition of the *Diagnostic and Statistical Manual*,[1] PTSD has 6 components **(Table 1)**.

This article first appeared in Clin Geriatr Med 2014;30(3):577–589.

Disclosure: This material is the result of work supported with resources and the use of facilities at the Boston VA Medical Center. Dr J. Moye received funding for research from the Department of Veterans Affairs Rehabilitation Research and Development Service #5I01RX000104-02. Conflict of Interest: The authors have no conflict of interest relating to this study or this article.

[a] VA Boston Health Care System, Brockton, MA, USA; [b] Department of Psychiatry, Harvard Medical School, MA, USA

* Corresponding author. Brockton Division, VA Boston Healthcare System, 940 Belmont Street, Brockton, MA 02301.

E-mail address: jennifer.moye@va.gov

Psychiatr Clin N Am 38 (2015) 45–57
http://dx.doi.org/10.1016/j.psc.2014.11.003
0193-953X/15/$ – see front matter Published by Elsevier Inc.

psych.theclinics.com

Table 1
Diagnostic criteria for PTSD

Criterion	Description
(A) Exposure	Event with actual or threatened death, serious injury, or sexual violation by: Directly experiencing the traumatic event Witnessing in person the traumatic event as it occurred to others Learning that the traumatic event occurred to a close family member/friend Experiencing first-hand repeated or extreme exposure to aversive details of the traumatic event
(B) Reexperiencing	Spontaneous memories of the traumatic event, recurrent distressing dreams, dissociative reactions, intense or prolonged psychological distress or physiologic reaction to cues
(C) Avoidance	Avoidance of distressing memories, thoughts, feelings, or external reminders of the event
(D) Negative cognitions and mood	Persistent and distorted negative beliefs about oneself, others, the world, or causes/consequences of traumatic event; persistent negative emotional state, diminished interest, detachment/estrangement from others; persistent inability to feel positive emotions; inability to remember key aspects of the event
(E) Arousal	Irritable/angry, reckless or self-destructive behavior, hypervigilance, exaggerated startle, problems with concentration or sleep
(F) Duration	More than 1 mo
(G) Functional impairment	Clinically significant distress or impairment in social, occupational, or other important areas of functioning

Risk Factors

Although studies vary as to whether age[2–4] increases risk for medically induced PTSD, several other factors are consistently associated with increased risk (**Box 1**).[2,4–6]

Scope of the Problem

Medically induced PTSD affects the individual, the family, and the health care system. Individuals with PTSD with comorbid depression experience more severe depression,[7] particularly intrusion symptoms, and all-cause mortality.[8] Family and professional caregivers may experience emotional distancing, irritability, and aggression from patients with PTSS,[9] and may also experience increased psychological distress themselves.[10] Older adults with PTSD may have more frequent primary care visits but not receive indicated mental health treatment.[11]

Box 1
Risk factors for medically induced PTSD

- Previous trauma or negative life stressors
- Preexisting psychiatric disorder
- Higher exposure to trauma (eg, longer intensive care unit [ICU] stay; longer duration of cancer treatment)
- Loss of physical functioning as a result of the medical condition
- Pain

Clinical Correlations

Many conditions are associated with risk of PTSD or PTSS (**Box 2**).

DIAGNOSTIC STANDARDS AND DILEMMAS
Process of Eliminating Alternative Diagnoses/Problems

Although anxiety and depression may frequently co-occur with catastrophic medical illness, PTSD can be differentiated from these, especially by the presence of experiences described by the patient as traumatic (criterion A) and intrusive thoughts, memories, and dreams of these events (criterion B). Avoidance is a cardinal component of PTSD but may not be present if the patient is unable to avoid aversive reminders (such as having to return for ongoing health care at the site of the initial diagnosis or subsequent procedures) and even because the body may be a daily reminder (eg, a missing breast). In addition, clinicians should remain alert for PTSS (ie, the presence of symptoms that do not meet criteria for the disorder but still cause clinically significant distress and dysfunction).

Comorbidities

Depression,[12] bipolar disorder,[13] and dementia can occur with PTSD; PTSD conveys an increased risk for developing dementia.[14,15] Although difficult medical experiences may lead to PTSD symptoms, older adults with lifetime PTSD have high rates of physical health conditions, such as of gastritis, angina pectoris, and arthritis.[16] Social changes such as retirement and bereavement may be associated with increased thoughts about military experience earlier in their lives.[17]

CLINICAL FINDINGS
Source of Data

Patient interview and reports of family and professional caregivers provide the key data on PTSD. Patients are most aware of internal signs and often do not tell others

---

Box 2
Conditions associated with medically induced PTSD and PTSD prevalence rates

Diagnoses of life-threatening illness

    Cancer, 0%–35%[34]

    Multiple sclerosis, 16%–75%[35]

Medical events

    Myocardial infarction, 5%[36]–42%[5,37]

    Stroke, 8%–9%[38]

    Delirium, 19%–22%[39]

    Fall, 17%–35%[3]

Surgical procedures

    Cardiac surgery, 17%–20%[40,41]

    Intraoperative awareness, 2%–71%[42,43]

Medical settings

    ICU, 10%–28%[44]

    Long-term care, 9%–22%[45]

about intrusive symptoms. Caregivers are often more aware of external signs such as anger and agitation.

Examination

A clinical interview focusing on symptoms of PTSD is the foundation of the examination. The most important issue is to ask about the occurrence and impact of catastrophic medical events because PTSSs from these are often overlooked. Begin by simply asking about the recent medical experience. For example: "You were recently hospitalized for heart surgery. How was that for you? Some people find themselves having bad memories or dreams of their heart surgery and recovery. Have you found that? Is there anything that happened you wish to discuss? Do you have any questions about your surgery and hospital stay?"

Recommended Rating Scales

Numerous self-report and interview measures can be used to guide PTSD assessment (**Table 2**). These instruments have been validated for use in older adults[18] and can be selected from factors such as brevity versus depth. A lower cut score of 42 (rather than 50) is recommended for older adults on the Posttraumatic Stress Disorder Check List.[19]

INTERVENTIONS: CURRENT EVIDENCE BASE AND WHAT TO DO WHEN EVIDENCE IS LACKING

Treatment of older adults with PTSD, particularly when medically induced, is weakly supported by age-specific and trigger-specific evidence. Although progress has been made on assessment and treatment protocols in the adult population, similar advances have lagged behind for older adults.[20] Therefore, clinical decision making must draw from the literature on younger adults and war or sexual trauma, supplemented with clinical experience.

Many older veterans whom we have seen in our practice at the Veteran's Administration have PTSD related to military trauma. Much of the research available for pharmacologic treatment is based on military-related PTSD or sexual trauma. However, our experience has shown us that elderly patients can have new-onset PTSD symptoms or exacerbation of previously remitted PTSD symptoms in the context of severe medical illness, and may benefit from similar treatment approaches. For example, a 66-year-old Vietnam-era combat veteran had remitted combat PTSD symptoms for

| Table 2 | | |
| Selected assessment scales | | |
Scale	Number of Items	Description
Primary Care PTSD Screen[46]	4	Designed to screen for PTSD in primary care and other medical settings, with an introductory sentence to cue respondents to traumatic events
Posttraumatic Check List–Stressor-specific version[47]	17	Severity rating of 17 PTSD symptoms in relation to a specific stressful experience
Impact of Events Scale - Revised[48]	22	Severity rating of subjective distress caused by traumatic events

many years. He was recently emergently hospitalized for a ventricular tachycardia after his implantable cardioverter defibrillator fired 5 consecutive times while he was alone at the local sanitation station. He sat alone in his vehicle, called 911, and waited to die. Since this retriggering event, the veteran has developed reemerging symptoms of PTSD including hyperarousal, anxiety, nightmares, depressed mood, and ruminative thoughts of death; these thoughts intermix with his earlier trauma and his memories of his cardiac event.

PSYCHOPHARMACOLOGIC TREATMENT

Pharmacologic interventions should target the individual core symptoms of PTSD with attention paid to the medical comorbidities and the risks and benefits of medications. As patients feel threatened, as in the case of the Vietnam veteran during and after his cardiac event, overwhelming fear tends to trigger a typical fight-or-flight response with symptoms of nightmares, insomnia, depressed and anxious mood, and hyperarousal, which is thought to arise from the brain's amygdala. Psychopharmacology in PTSD is focused on restoring balance to the natural inhibitory response of the brain. At present, the US Food and Drug Administration (FDA) has approved only 2 medications for PTSD: the selective serotonin reuptake inhibitors (SSRIs), paroxetine and sertraline. There is currently much research in progress to assess whether these medications are the best available choices for PTSD symptoms. However, first it may be helpful to discuss the use of benzodiazepines, which are widely prescribed for PTSD in medical settings.

Benzodiazepines

Gamma-aminobutyric acid (GABA) is an inhibitory neurotransmitter that, when activated by benzodiazepines (BZDs), is decreases neuronal firing and anxiety. Many clinicians immediately prescribe these drugs without concern for their effects. BZDs can be effective in treating symptoms of anxiety disorders including PTSD and are usually safe. However, in the geriatric population, there are many reasons why these drugs are heavily regulated. Even the BZDs with shorter half-lives (such as alprazolam and lorazepam) must be used with caution in older adults, because of the potential for increased half-life caused by slower hepatic metabolism and decreased renal clearance.[21] Comorbid medical illnesses (cancer, renal and kidney disease, dementia, cardiac disease, vascular disorders) increase risks for adverse drug effects such as gait impairment, falls, confusion, and psychomotor slowing, and intentional or unwitting overuse can also increase risk for motor vehicle and other accidents and unsafe behaviors. Risks of dependency, tolerance, delirium, and withdrawal are also a concern. For all these reasons, BZDs should not be considered drugs of choice in treatment of PTSD, and are best reserved as a last resort.

PREFERRED PHARMACOLOGIC MANAGEMENT OF PTSD SYMPTOMS
Sleep

Patients often report that insomnia is the most distressing PTSD symptom. Lack of sleep can exacerbate other symptoms of PTSD. For these reasons it is useful to treat insomnia first.[22] Sleep disturbances in PTSD are thought to be related to hyperarousal and increased adrenergic activity, which may lead to related symptoms such as nightmares, difficulty initiating sleep, and frequent awakenings. Two medications that decrease nightmares and improve sleep quality are prazosin, and trazodone.[23]

In elderly populations, prazosin (an alpha-1 adrenergic receptor antagonist that crosses blood-brain barrier) is effective but risks of postural hypotension, dizziness, and priapism should be monitored. Risks can be minimized by starting at the lowest possible dosage and titrating slowly. Low-dose trazodone (with activity at 5HT2A, alpha 1, and H1 receptors) is an alternative to prazosin and may help with sleep onset. Because of alpha 1 activity, it also can cause postural hypotension and priapism, especially in combination with prazosin, and patients should be monitored closely. Other medications for sleep include tricyclic antidepressants or sedating atypical antipsychotics (quetiapine). However, a careful individualized review of risks versus benefits is necessary when considering these medications in the elderly.

Hyperarousal, Avoidance, and Reexperiencing

If prazosin and or trazodone are ineffective in treating all the symptoms of PTSD, the next step is to consider a trial of an SSRI. The choice of an antidepressant is crucial. Elderly patients are often nonadherant to medications[24] for several reasons including worry over adverse side effects, costs of medications, fear of addiction, and lack of understanding of the value of medications. Clinical response improves with adherence so when discussing risks and benefits of individual medications with patients there should be clear communication about the patients' conflicting beliefs and preconceived ideas. Addressing these concerns may improve overall compliance. Open communication related to particular side effects of antidepressants can improve knowledge and expectations about the medication in the patient, and thus improve adherence For example, choosing paroxetine (Paxil) for an 85-year-old man already taking oxybutynin for bladder incontinence may potentiate anticholinergic symptoms of dry mouth, sedation, confusion, and ataxia, thus causing the patient to stop the medication prematurely or become delirious. Monitoring comorbid medical conditions, prescribed and nonprescribed over-the-counter medications, as well as having specific target symptoms (sleep, appetite, nightmares, and anxiety) can make this process smoother.

Psychosis

Some geriatric patients experience psychotic symptoms associated with PTSD. In our experience, this is more likely to be the case when PTSD occurs in combination with dementia, and dementia can reveal quiescent PTSD from decades earlier. Low-dose quetiapine, risperidone, and aripiprazole may be helpful in reducing or eliminating psychotic symptoms. The benefits of these medications must be weighed against the risks of side effects such as weight gain, metabolic syndrome, and cardiovascular risk.

As with all psychiatric medications used in older adults, it is important to start low and go slow, but go. More cautious titration usually results in better tolerance. In contrast, excessive caution can result in failure to reach a therapeutic dose of medication and limited treatment benefit as well as loss of patient confidence resulting in noncompliance. Educate the patient that symptoms can take up to 6 weeks to remit and that consistency of dosing and clinician contact are important in achieving the best results. If the first medication yields only partial response, consider increasing the dosage, augmenting with a second agent, or switching to another medication (**Table 3**).

NONPHARMACOLOGIC TREATMENT
Lifespan Context

In work with older veterans who are experiencing PTSD, often as a resurgence of symptoms late in life, the decision of whether and how to approach the trauma narrative is tempered by the combat trauma having occurred 40 to 60 years ago, being

Table 3
Medications for PTSD

Medication	Target	Notable Side Effects	Geriatric Considerations
First-line Treatment			
Prazosin 1–6 mg PO QHS Titrate by 1 mg weekly until effect or side effects	Hyperarousal Nightmares Fragmented sleep	Orthostatic hypotension Dizziness Headache Slowed heart rate Priapism if taken with trazodone	May only need small dose. (1–3 mg) Titrate cautiously Consider changing BP medication to prazosin Monitor blood pressure or falls
Trazodone 12.5–100 mg PO QHS Titrate by 12.5–25 mg weekly		As for prazosin, and also sedation	Affects serotonin and histamine, and blocks alpha-adrenergic receptors Avoid aggressive dosing
SSRIs in Order of Choice			
Escitalopram 5–10 mg PO daily	Hyperarousal Reexperiencing Depressed mood Sleep disturbance	Sexual side effects Low sodium levels (rare) Usually well tolerated (fewer GI symptoms)	Most effective of the SSRIs Active enantiomer of citalopram; risk for QTC prolongation is lower at dosages of 5–10 mg daily than with equivalent citalopram dose of 20–40 mg Usually well tolerated
Sertraline 12.5–100 mg PO daily Titrate by 12.5 weekly		Diarrhea/nausea Sedation Sexual side effects Hyponatremia (rare)	More effective in women If GI symptoms do not remit, consider change in medication If sedated during the day, switch time of medication to QHS
Fluoxetine 5–40 mg PO daily Titrate by 5 mg every other week		Diarrhea/nausea Sleep interference Potentiates anticoagulants	Many drug-drug interactions caused by CYP450 enzyme system Long half-life Not usually beneficial in elderly patients with PTSD
SNRIs as Next Line of Treatment in Order of Choice			
Venlafaxine SA 37.5–150 mg PO daily Titrate by 37.5 mg every 7–14 d until effect	Depressed mood Avoidance No benefit for insomnia, hyperarousal	Can increase hyperarousal because of noradrenergic activation Hypertension Monitor liver function tests	Reasonable second-line treatment when SSRIs fail SA formula usually better tolerated Discontinuation syndrome: needs slow taper if ineffective

(continued on next page)

Table 3 (continued)			
Medication	**Target**	**Notable Side Effects**	**Geriatric Considerations**
Mirtazapine 7.5–30 mg QHS Titrate by 7.5 mg weekly	Hyperarousal Anxiety Depressed mood Sleep onset	Postural hypotension Dizziness Weight gain Low WBC (rare)	Good choice for cachectic, ill patients if able to tolerate risk of hypotension
Bupropion SR 100–300 mg PO daily Start 100 mg daily for 7 d then increase to 100 mg BID	Fatigue Depressed mood Avoidance	Can cause greater hyperarousal May interfere with sleep	May use with trazodone and or prazosin No sexual side effects, which may be an advantage to some patients Needs more study for PTSD

Abbreviations: BID, twice a day; BP, blood pressure; CYP450, cytochrome P 450; GI, gastrointestinal; PO, orally; QHS, at bedtime; SNRI, serotonin-norepinephrine reuptake inhibitor; WBC, white blood cell count.

interwoven with that individual's lifespan development, and occurring in the context of multiple vulnerabilities such as chronic illness and, potentially, lower cognitive resources. Our research on older veteran cancer survivors suggests a different approach to PTSD symptoms when they arise out of catastrophic medical events rather than war or sexual trauma. We find that younger old veterans (eg, ages 55–65 years) are more likely than older veterans to experience PTSD arising out of the diagnosis and treatment of cancer, and that those with concurrent combat PTSD symptoms are at increased risk for cancer-related PTSD.[25] Older veterans (eg, ages 75–85 years) seem less likely to develop PTSD arising out of medical experience, which may be because of resilience acquired through facing other health and emotional challenges in late life and different normative expectations related to age. These contextual factors influence how we approach the treatment of PTSD symptoms arising out of late-life medical experience.

Eliciting the Trauma Narrative

As with psychopharmacologic treatment, psychotherapy can be used to target specific core symptom groups of PTSD, particularly reexperiencing, numbing, and hyperarousal. Intrusive thoughts, memories, and nightmares are often a signal to patients, families, and health care providers that an individual is having PTSD symptoms that may benefit from treatment. A common starting place in PTSD treatment with psychotherapeutic approaches such as prolonged exposure and cognitive processing therapy (CPT) is a telling and retelling of the trauma story, which individuals often keep to themselves. The telling of the trauma narrative serves several purposes. First, because memory processing during traumatic events is likely to be interrupted, it allows the individual to reconstruct a set of possibly fragmented memories into a coherent narrative from which to build meaning. Second, it desensitizes the individual's psychological and psychophysiologic reaction to the memories as a conditioned stimulus that elicits a fear response, in hopes that it will allow the individual to put less energy into avoiding these and the difficulties that can come with the processes of avoidance. In addition, the process of sharing and allowing another person to bear witness decreases the profound isolation that often accompanies traumatic experience. In contrast with eliciting a combat trauma narrative, our experience is that there is less fragmentation of the memories than commonly occurs in combat and sexual trauma, but, at times, more embarrassment and isolation when the trauma is medical in nature.

Reducing Isolation

The therapeutic process of eliciting and sharing stressful or traumatic medical experiences seems to be useful in reducing intrusive memories and dreams, as well as the numbing symptoms of PTSD, in this case particularly the withdrawal from others. It is our experience that health care providers can become accustomed or sometimes desensitized to the felt responses of patients when performing procedures repeatedly, and that patients, grateful for their care, are reluctant to complain. Because of this, patients may feel alone. For example, some veterans have shared with us that treatments for urologic cancers involved moments of profound embarrassment, fear, or pain (eg, external beam radiation to the prostate, surveillance cystoscopies), all the more so if the veteran has experienced combat trauma as well as childhood sexual trauma.[26] In our clinic's cancer support group, a key intervention is for veterans to be able to share their experiences of treatments and surveillance procedures. In this case, companionship with others who are having similar experiences greatly reduces the burden of isolation, and it is hoped that this will extend to other relationships outside the group.

Managing Hyperarousal

In addition, individual or group psychotherapy can target management of PTSD symptoms of hyperarousal. For example, many cancer survivors find that surveillance imaging causes anxious arousal. Again, this can be worsened in the context of combat trauma. For example, a young veteran has shared that the process of being tied into a magnetic resonance imaging (MRI) cage and placed into an MRI scanner can elicit memories of target searching of tunnels in Vietnam. He finds it useful to ask other veterans to accompany him to scan appointments and to use a combination of benzodiazepine and antihistamine for symptom management. As another example, an older veteran has shared that surveillance scans remind him of hiding beneath floor boards in a French farm house behind German lines, as Germans searched the house. This veteran shared that he approaches scans by clenching his fists and imagining that the MRI sounds are combat sounds, which, for him, provides more mastery than focusing on the present moment. Therefore, in both individual and group psychotherapy it is useful to discuss upcoming medical appointments and procedures, to ensure that the patient is not avoiding these, and also to develop strategies for normalizing and managing any anxiety that may arise. It can also be useful to directly communicate these issues to other health care providers (with the patient's permission) or coach the patient in how to address these with providers (eg, radiology technicians).

Assuaging Worry

However, there are some differences in the psychotherapeutic treatment of PTSD symptoms arising from combat compared with catastrophic or threatening medical experience. The treatment of combat PTSD symptoms focuses on the experiences of combat and how these have, and are, affecting a person's life. The treatment of medical PTSD symptoms may be less retrospective, involving less narrative reconstruction, but more prospective, involving consideration of disease management going forward. For example, for many, a core psychological component is fear of recurrence.[27] In our research we have also found that cancer survivors have other significant worries, including worries about the burden of the disease on family (eg, "Who will take care of my family when I'm gone?"), about long-term side effects (eg, "When will I start to feel better?"), and existential issues (eg, "Am I making the most of the time

I have?").[27] Therefore psychotherapeutic treatment of cancer-related PTSD is likely to involve strategies for managing worries; for example, through mindfulness or acceptance techniques. As an example, in our cancer support group, if a veteran describes getting a worrisome test result, another veteran often reintroduces the idea of waiting to get the information and then making a plan 1 day at a time.

Working from strengths (resilience developed in facing past traumas) is an important component of treating PTSD in older veterans. Posttraumatic growth, the perception of positive benefits arising from trauma, may moderate the association between PTSD symptoms and mental health outcomes following cardiac surgery.[28]

EARLY INTERVENTION

PTSD arising out of medical trauma occurs in or near a health care context, providing the opportunity for early intervention by health care providers. Although early trauma debriefing is not advised,[29] more recent approaches have combined early intervention in the inpatient setting, supplemented with pharmacotherapy and psychotherapy in the weeks after discharge, a so-called stepped collaborative care approach, to reduce PTSD symptoms.[30] Although not tested in older adults, these and other early intervention strategies involving medication[31] or psychotherapy[32] in the acute stage of trauma hold much promise.[33] For example, falling is a common problem in older adults, and is associated with subsequent PTSD symptoms and fear of falling.[3] Screening and early intervention in the emergency or hospital setting could potentially prevent the excess morbidity caused by activity restriction, although these outcomes need to be studied.

Knowledge Needs for Health Care Improvement Going Forward

Although the literature has ample reports of PTSD related to catastrophic medical diagnosis and treatments, and considerable data on the treatment of sexual or combat PTSD, it lacks adequate theoretic and outcome studies of treatment of PTSD in older adults, and there is almost no information about special considerations in treating PTSD arising out of medical experience in older adults. Randomized treatment trials of psychopharmacologic and/or psychotherapeutic approaches to reducing PTSD symptoms are needed, but so are qualitative studies that systematically describe the varieties of PTSD symptoms that develop after accidents, injuries, and medical illness in older patients. In addition, further inquiry into the role of the health care team in recognition; early intervention; and, in situations in which medical events and care can traumatize patients, prevention is also badly needed.

REFERENCES

1. American Psychiatric Association. Diagnostic and statistical manual of mental disorders. 5th edition. Arlington (VA): American Psychiatric Association; 2013.
2. Boer KR, van Ruler O, Emmerik AA, et al. Factors associated with posttraumatic stress symptoms in a prospective cohort of patients after abdominal sepsis: a nomogram. Intensive Care Med 2008;34(4):664–74.
3. Man Cheung C, McKee KJ, Austin C, et al. Posttraumatic stress disorder in older people after a fall. Int J Geriatr Psychiatry 2009;24(9):955–64.
4. Whitehead DL, Perkins-Porras L, Strike PC, et al. Post-traumatic stress disorder in patients with cardiac disease: predicting vulnerability from emotional responses during admission for acute coronary syndromes. Heart 2006;92(9):1225–9.
5. Wilder Schaaf KP, Artman LK, Peberdy MA, et al. Anxiety, depression, and PTSD following cardiac arrest: a systematic review of the literature. Resuscitation 2013; 84:873–7.

6. French-Rosas L, Moye J, Naik A. Improving the recognition and treatment of cancer-related posttraumatic stress disorder. J Psychiatr Pract 2011;17:270–6.
7. Chan D, Fan MY, Unützer J. Long-term effectiveness of collaborative depression care in older primary care patients with and without PTSD symptoms. Int J Geriatr Psychiatry 2011;26(7):758–64.
8. Edmondson D, Rieckmann N, Shaffer JA, et al. Posttraumatic stress due to an acute coronary syndrome increases risk of 42-month major adverse cardiac events and all-cause mortality. J Psychiatr Res 2011;45(12):1621–6.
9. So SS, La Guardia JG. Matters of the heart: patients' adjustment to life following a cardiac crisis. Psychol Health 2011;26:83–100.
10. Bunzel B, Roethy W, Znoj H, et al. Psychological consequences of life-saving cardiac surgery in patients and partners: measurement of emotional stress by the impact of event scale. Stress Health 2008;24(5):351–63.
11. Van Zelst WH, De Beurs E, Beekman AT, et al. Well-being, physical functioning, and use of health services in the elderly with PTSD and subthreshold PTSD. Int J Geriatr Psychiatry 2006;21(2):180–8.
12. Ginzburg K. Comorbidity of PTSD and depression following myocardial infarction. J Affect Disord 2006;94(1–3):135–43.
13. Sajatovic M, Blow FC, Ignacio RV. Psychiatric comorbidity in older adults with bipolar disorder. Int J Geriatr Psychiatry 2006;21(6):582–7.
14. Qureshi SU, Kimbrell T, Pyne JM, et al. Greater prevalence and incidence of dementia in older veterans with posttraumatic stress disorder. J Am Geriatr Soc 2010;58(9):1627–33.
15. Kristine Yaffe K, Vittinghoff E, Lindquist K, et al. Posttraumatic stress disorder and risk of dementia among US veterans. Arch Gen Psychiatry 2010;67:608–13.
16. Pietrzak RH, Goldstein RB, Southwick SM, et al. Physical health conditions associated with posttraumatic stress disorder in U.S. older adults: results from wave 2 of the National Epidemiologic Survey on Alcohol and Related Conditions. J Am Geriatr Soc 2012;60(2):296–303.
17. Davison EH, Pless AP, Gugliucci MR, et al. Late-life emergence of early-life trauma. Res Aging 2006;28(1):84–114.
18. Thorp SR, Sones HM, Cook JM. Posttraumatic stress disorder among older adults. In: Sorocco KH, Lauderdale S, editors. Cognitive behavior therapy with older adults: innovations across care settings. New York: Springer Publishing Company; 2011. p. 189–218.
19. Cook JM, Thompson R, Coyne JC, et al. Algorithm versus cut-point derived PTSD in ex-prisoners of war. J Psychopathol Behav Assess 2003;25:267–71.
20. Cook JM, O'Donnell C. Assessment and psychological treatment of posttraumatic stress disorder in older adults. J Geriatr Psychiatry Neurol 2005;18(2):61–71.
21. Salzman C. Clinical geriatric psychopharmacology. Philadelphia: Lippincott Williams & Wilkins; 2005.
22. Bajor LA, Ticlea AN, Osser DN. Psychopharmacology Algorithm Project at the Harvard South Shore program: an update on PTSD. Harv Rev Psychiatry 2011;19:240–58.
23. Stahl SM. Stahl's essential psychopharmacology. 3rd edition. New York: Cambridge University Press; 2009.
24. Vik SA, Maxwell CJ, Hogan DB. Measurement, correlates, and health outcomes of medication adherence among seniors. Ann Pharmacother 2004;38:303–12.
25. Moye J, Gosian J, Snow R, et al, Vetcares Research Team. Emotional health following diagnosis and treatment of oral-digestive cancer in military veterans.

119th Annual Meeting of the American Psychological Association. Washington, DC, August 4–7, 2011.

26. Hilgeman M, Moye J, Archambault E, et al. In the veterans voice. Fed Pract 2012; 29(Suppl):51S–9S.

27. Moye J, Wachen JS, Mulligan EA, et al. Assessing multidimensional worry in cancer survivors. Psychooncology 2014;23:237–40.

28. Bluvstein I, Moravchick L, Sheps D, et al. Posttraumatic growth, posttraumatic stress symptoms and mental health among coronary heart disease survivors. J Clin Psychol Med Settings 2013;20(2):164–72.

29. Rose S, Bisson J, Churchill R, et al. Psychological debriefing for preventing post traumatic stress disorder (PTSD). Cochrane Database Syst Rev 2002;(2):CD000560.

30. Zatzick D, Roy-Byrne P, Russo J, et al. A randomized effectiveness trial of stepped collaborative care for acutely injured trauma survivors. Arch Gen Psychiatry 2004;61:498–506.

31. Schelling G, Roozendaal B, Krauseneck T, et al. Efficacy of hydrocortisone in preventing posttraumatic stress disorder following critical illness and major surgery. Ann N Y Acad Sci 2006;1071:46–53.

32. Rothbaum BO, Houry D, Heekin M, et al. A pilot study of an exposure-based intervention in the ED designed to prevent posttraumatic stress disorder. Am J Emerg Med 2008;26:326–30.

33. Kearns MC, Ressler KJ, Zatzick D, et al. Early interventions for PTSD: a review. Depress Anxiety 2012;29:833–42.

34. Kangas M, Henry JL, Bryant RA. Posttraumatic stress disorder following cancer: a conceptual and empirical review. Clin Psychol Rev 2002;22(4):499–524.

35. Chalfant AM, Bryant RA, Fulcher G. Posttraumatic stress disorder following diagnosis of multiple sclerosis. J Trauma Stress 2004;17(5):423–8.

36. O'Reilly SM, Grubb N, O'Carroll RE. Long-term emotional consequences of in-hospital cardiac arrest and myocardial infarction. Br J Clin Psychol 2004;43(1): 83–95.

37. Chung MC, Berger Z, Jones R, et al. Posttraumatic stress and co-morbidity following myocardial infarction among older patients: the role of coping. Aging Ment Health 2008;12(1):124–33.

38. Sembi S, Tarrier N, O'Neill P, et al. Does post-traumatic stress disorder occur after stroke: a preliminary study. Int J Geriatr Psychiatry 1998;13(5):315–22.

39. Dimartini A, Dew MA, Kormos R, et al. Posttraumatic stress disorder caused by hallucinations and delusions experienced in delirium. Psychosomatics 2007;48: 436–9.

40. Parmigiani G, Tarsitani L, De Santis V, et al. Attachment style and posttraumatic stress disorder after cardiac surgery. Eur Psychiatry 2013;28:S1.

41. Rothenhäusler HB, Stepan A. The effects of cardiac surgery on health-related quality of life, and emotional status outcomes: a follow-up study. Eur Psychiatry 2010;25:515.

42. Bruchas R, Kent C, Wilson H, et al. Anesthesia awareness: narrative review of psychological sequelae, treatment, and incidence. J Clin Psychol Med Settings 2011;18(3):257–67.

43. Mashour GA, Wang LY, Turner CR, et al. A retrospective study of intraoperative awareness with methodological implications. Anesth Analg 2009;108:521–6.

44. Davydow DS, Gifford JM, Desai SV, et al. Posttraumatic stress disorder in general intensive care unit survivors: a systematic review. Gen Hosp Psychiatry 2008;30: 421–34.

45. Carlson EB, Lauderdale S, Hawkins J, et al. Posttraumatic stress and aggression among veterans in long-term care. J Geriatr Psychiatry Neurol 2008;21(1):61–71.
46. Prins A, Ouimette P, Kimerling R, et al. The primary care PTSD screen (PC-PTSD): development and operating characteristics. Prim Care Psychiatr 2004;9(1):9–14.
47. Weathers FW, Litz BT, Herman DS, et al. The PTSD checklist (PCL-C): reliability, validity, and diagnostic utility. Annual Convention of the International Society for Traumatic Stress Studies. San Antonio (TX), November, 1993.
48. Weiss DS, Marmar CR. The impact of event scale - revised. In: Keane JW, editor. Assessing psychological trauma and PTSD. New York: Guilford; 1996. p. 399–411.

The Interface of Child Mental Health and Juvenile Diabetes Mellitus

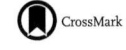

Sandra L. Fritsch, MD[a,b],*, Mark W. Overton, MD[c],
Douglas R. Robbins, MD[a,d,e]

KEYWORDS

- Diabetes mellitus • Children • Adolescents • Psychosocial functioning
- Cognitive functioning • Mental health

Diabetes mellitus (type 1) has long been identified as one of the most common chronic, lifelong illnesses developing in childhood. In the United States, type 2 diabetes and metabolic syndrome are increasing in children and adolescents at an alarming rate.[1,2] Type 1 diabetes mellitus (T1DM) has also been called insulin-dependent diabetes mellitus (IDDM) and juvenile onset diabetes mellitus. The hallmark feature of T1DM is the under production or lack of production of insulin by the beta cells of the pancreas. This lack of insulin is felt to be due to the destruction of the beta cells. The hallmark feature of type 2 diabetes is "insulin resistance." In type 2 diabetes, the pancreatic beta cells still make insulin, but cells become "resistant" to insulin and are unable to take up circulating glucose. Thus, high levels of circulating insulin and glucose are found in type 2 diabetes.[3] Risk factors for type 2 diabetes include being overweight (**Table 1**). The incidence of overweight children and adolescents (above the 95th percentile for weight) has been increasing during the last few decades, with 17.1% of all children and adolescents being defined as overweight in 2003 and 2004.[4,5] Risk factors for children and adolescents becoming overweight and who are at risk for metabolic syndrome or type 2 diabetes have

This article first appeared in Child and Adolescent Psychiatric Clinics N Am 2011;19(2), and also appeared in Pediatr Clin N Am 2011;58:937–54.

[a] Child and Adolescent Psychiatry, Maine Medical Center, Tufts University School of Medicine, 22 Bramhall Street, Portland, ME 04102, USA; [b] Department of Psychiatry, Child & Adolescent Psychiatry Fellowship, Maine Medical Center, 22 Bramhall Street, Portland, ME 04102, USA; [c] Northern Maine Medical Center, Fort Kent 04743, ME, USA; [d] Department of Psychiatry, The Glickman Family Center for Child & Adolescent Psychiatry, Maine Medical Center, 22 Bramhall Street, Portland, ME 04102, USA; [e] Department of Psychiatry, Child & Adolescent Psychiatry, Maine Medical Center, 22 Bramhall Street, Portland, ME 04102, USA

* Corresponding author. Department of Psychiatry, Child & Adolescent Psychiatry Fellowship, Maine Medical Center, 22 Bramhall Street, Portland, ME 04102.
E-mail address: fritss@mmc.org

Table 1
Differences among T1DM, type 2 diabetes mellitus, and metabolic syndrome

Type 1 Diabetes Mellitus	Type 2 Diabetes Mellitus	Metabolic Syndrome
Onset: abrupt; often in childhood Insulin dependent Defect: insulin producing cells of the pancreas	Onset: gradual; originally adult disease, now increasing in childhood Insulin resistant: hallmark feature Associated with obesity, use of atypical antipsychotic medications May be controlled with diet and exercise	Constellation of symptoms including: ■ Abdominal adiposity ■ Elevated triglycerides ■ Low HDL ■ Hypertension ■ Type 2 diabetes may be associated Risk for cardiovascular disease May be associated with use of atypical antipsychotic medications

included the increased use of atypical antipsychotics, most notably olanzapine and clozapine.[6–9]

The incidence of T1DM varies with geography, age, gender, family history, and race. Risk for developing T1DM in childhood seems to increase with distance from the equator.[10] In the United States, the highest incidence of T1DM is found in non-Hispanic white children, 23.6 per 100,000 annually.[11] Childhood-onset T1DM has a bimodal presentation for age of onset, with the first peak between ages 4 and 6 years and the second peak in early adolescence.[12]

Development of childhood-onset IDDM occurs with the destruction of the beta cells in the pancreas. The destruction is most often felt to be mediated by an autoimmune response but can also be seen in association with cystic fibrosis. In addition, there is noted genetic susceptibility as the risk for T1DM increases for first-degree relatives.[13] Thus, for genetically susceptible individuals, it is postulated that environmental exposures (proposed agents including: viral infections, immunizations, diet, vitamin D deficiency and perinatal factors) trigger an immune response, leading to the destruction of the beta cells of the pancreas. There is also an associated increased risk for celiac disease for children with T1DM. Some children and families struggle with the dietary restrictions of T1DM and the gluten-free dietary requirements for celiac disease.

The treatment regimen for T1DM includes close monitoring of blood glucose level by "finger sticks," monitoring of urine for glycosuria, diet modifications, and multiple injections of insulin per day. Some treatment centers advocate "tight" control, with blood glucose levels monitored as frequently as every 4 hours and decisions on insulin dose made as predicated by the blood glucose level. Other programs may have as "loose" a program as twice a day injections and twice a day monitoring of blood and urine glucose levels. But in the developing child with variable times of exercise, school lunches, birthday parties ensuring healthy blood glucose levels can be a challenge to the child, the family, and the care providers. Often in later adolescence, the individual with T1DM may opt (or be recommended by the treatment provider) to receive treatment from an insulin pump (subcutaneous continuous infusion of insulin). The insulin pump delivers continuous basal insulin with boluses associated with meals. Use of the insulin pump may reduce rates of hypoglycemic events, but controlled trials of pump therapy comparing injection therapy in the pediatric population are currently limited.[14,15]

There are both long-term complications of chronically high blood glucose levels on the vascular system and serious short-term problems with acute hypoglycemic events

(**Box 1**). The preschool-age child may be more vulnerable to severe hypoglycemic events, and prepubertal children may be more protected from microvascular complications of T1DM. For the person with frequent "sugars running high," measurement of the glycated hemoglobin levels (A_{1c}) will be elevated. The recognized risk of hypoglycemia in younger children has led to the setting of higher HbA_{1c} target levels compared with the expectation of "stricter" metabolic control for older children and adolescents.

Shorter-term complications of diabetes include difficulties associated with hypoglycemia, ranging from tremor, confusion, and lethargy to stupor and seizures. Acute hyperglycemia can lead to polyuria, nocturnal enuresis, weight loss, and risk for diabetic ketoacidosis, which can potentially cause coma and death. Thus, diabetes can cause acute life-threatening events in addition to chronic complications. For the developing child and adolescent, effects of hypoglycemic events and hyperglycemia may cause cognition and neurodevelopmental challenges (see next section).

Longer-term complications of diabetes affect all organ systems, with the causal agent being microvascular damage. Most notable potential complications include retinopathy, nephropathy, neuropathy, cardiovascular disease, and impotence. Additional complications can include gastroparesis, menstrual difficulties, necrobiosis lipoidica, and bone changes.

EFFECT ON COGNITION AND NEUROPSYCHOLOGICAL DIFFICULTIES IN CHILDREN AND ADOLESCENTS

Children and adolescent brains continue to develop through pruning, myelinization, and other maturational processes. Childhood cognitive development is well recognized to undergo remarkable changes from barely recognizing letters to abstract thinking. The effect of hypoglycemia and hyperglycemia in the developing child on cognitive functioning and subtle neuropsychological deficits has been the subject of ongoing studies. In 2004, Desrocher and Rovet[16] provided a comprehensive review of the literature, some of the controversies, and a discussion of some of the limitations of past research. Further research since 2004 is described in the next section and in **Table 2**.

Hypoglycemia

Earlier age of onset (<5 years) has often been associated with more frequent or more severe bouts of hypoglycemia. This is thought to be secondary to individual lack of

Box 1 Complications of T1DM	
Short-term	*Long-term*
Hypoglycemia	Retinopathy
Confusion	Microvascular disease
Seizures	Nephropathy
Hyperglycemia	Neuropathy
Externalizing behaviors	Pregnancy complications
Diabetic ketoacidosis	Impotence
Coma	

Table 2
Long-term and immediate neurocognitive effects of hypoglycemia and hyperglycemia

	Hypoglycemia	Hyperglycemia
Long-term	■ Worse cognitive outcome ■ Decreased spatial intelligence ■ Delayed recall ■ Lower gray volume in left superior temporal region	■ Decreased verbal intelligence ■ Decreased gray volume in right cuneus and precuneus, smaller white volume in right posterior parietal region, increased gray matter in prefrontal region
Immediate	■ Problems with "selective attention" ■ Neuronal integrity in anterior brain seems susceptible to acute hypoglycemia	■ Increased externalizing behaviors ■ Susceptibility to cerebral edema in the frontal region associated with increased taurine

hypoglycemia awareness (or lack of verbal skills to express the acute event) and sensitivity to nocturnal hypoglycemic spells. Repeated severe bouts of hypoglycemia (more than 3 episodes) have been associated with deficits in spatial memory,[17] worse cognitive outcome and delayed recall,[18] and smaller gray matter volume in the left superior temporal region.[19] Greater exposure to severe hypoglycemia in childhood has also been associated with greater hippocampal volume,[20] and researchers postulated that this enlargement may reflect a pathologic reaction, leading to gliosis, reactive neurogenesis, or impairment of normal pruning.

A recent small study[21] tried to examine the immediate neuropsychological and neurometabolic effects of a severe hypoglycemic event (with associated seizure) in 3 prepubertal children. Immediate difficulties were noted with selective attention that improved during the subsequent 6 months, and the neuronal integrity in the anterior brain appeared particularly susceptible to acute hypoglycemia.

Hyperglycemia

Longer-term effects of chronic hyperglycemia have been noted to affect overall verbal intelligence,[18] overall brain changes including decreased gray matter volume in the right cuneus and precuneus regions, smaller white volume in the right posterior parietal region, and increased gray matter in the prefrontal region.[19]

Parents and children alike have anecdotally reported knowing when the child is running "high" glucoses by reporting changes in behavior. McDonnell and colleagues[22] studied prepubertal children with T1DM to test the potential association between glucose levels and behaviors. They, indeed, found an association between intercurrent high glycemic levels and increased externalizing behaviors, such as agitation and aggression. A recent study[23] conducted imaging studies during hyperglycemia in children with or without associated diabetic ketoacidosis, and the frontal region was notably affected with elevations of taurine associated with increased risk for cerebral edema.

Summary of Neurocognitive Effects of T1DM

T1DM has significant acute and chronic implications for the developing child and adolescent brain. Severe hypoglycemic episodes for children less than 5 years of age may later predispose the child to significant learning issues. On the other hand, chronically elevated glucose levels may predispose the child to lower verbal intelligence scores. Immediate effects of hypoglycemia may lead to problems with selective attention, whereas the child with "high sugars" may exhibit problematic externalizing behaviors. The child or adolescent and her/his family face the challenge of finding a correct balance.

PSYCHIATRIC COMORBIDITY ASSOCIATED WITH IDDM

Evidence suggests that maladjustment in children negatively affects glycemic control and subsequent metabolic functioning. Recent studies indicate elevated rates of psychiatric disorder between 33% and 42% in adolescents and young adults with diabetes,[24-26] which are 2 to 3 times higher than those found in the general population.[27-31] Diagnoses include internalizing and externalizing disorders. A recent study examined the effect of internalizing and externalizing disorders on the risk for readmission to the hospital for diabetes care, demonstrating an increased risk for readmission for adolescents (but not children) with internalizing behaviors and possibly an increased risk among those with externalizing behaviors.[32] Many studies suggest that individuals with comorbid psychiatric disorders are less likely to adhere to treatment regimens, resulting in poorer control of the illness.[30] Thus, disturbed adolescents with diabetes may be at "double jeopardy" for adverse physical and mental health outcomes.[30] An association between mood disorders in the child or adolescent with T1DM and family conflict and very "tight" metabolic control has also been reported,[33-35] raising the possibility that psychiatric symptoms may either contribute to or result from obsessive preoccupation with the demands of the diabetes treatment regimen.[30] Depression and anxiety are most commonly seen in children and adolescents with diabetes, and early adjustment disorders are more predictive of these diagnoses. Eating disorders are also common, particularly among women, and are discussed in the later section.

Adjustment Disorders

From the time of diagnosis, there is an expected pattern of adjustment because both children and families are introduced to a new world filled with challenges, constraints, and uncertainties associated with a lifelong illness. Initial adjustment to the diagnosis of diabetes is characterized by sadness, anxiety, withdrawal, and dependency,[36-39] and approximately 30% of children develop a clinical adjustment disorder in the 3 months subsequent to diagnosis.[36,40] Such difficulties often resolve within the first year, but poor adaptation in this initial phase places children at risk of later psychological difficulties.[26,30,36,38,41,42]

Depression

Studies have associated a diagnosis of depression with substantially worse glycemic control and more serious retinopathy in patients without psychiatric disorders.[43-45] Because of the overlap of symptoms such as fatigue, weight loss, and impaired memory common to both mood disorder and poor metabolic control, depression may be under diagnosed in children with diabetes.[36,43] Therefore, it is useful to reevaluate patients with symptoms of depression after glycemic control has been established. If symptoms persist, a diagnosis of depression may be indicated. Massengale[46] provides a recent review on the salient features of depression in the adolescent with T1DM. A 2003 study[47] reported that there is a 10-fold increase in the incidence of suicide and suicidal ideation in the adolescent with diabetes. In addition to other means, insulin is a potential means for self-injury.[48,49]

    With nearly one-third of diabetic adolescents experiencing comorbid depression and similar numbers reported in the adult population, researchers are looking for links of brain pathology/changes caused by the illness leading to increased risk for depression. McEwen and colleagues[50] propose that the progressive atrophy of the hippocampus is seen in animals with diabetes, which is similar to changes seen in depression.

Psychotherapeutic and psychopharmacologic interventions have been found to be helpful in treating depression. Psychopharmacologic treatment should be accompanied by psychotherapy addressing the pessimistic attitudes that typically accompany depression in adolescents and that can limit the patient's willingness or ability to do what is necessary to treat the diabetes.[43]

Psychopharmacologic treatment use in conjunction with IDDM may present with unique challenges. Although the initiation of treatment with antidepressants does not usually cause serious problems, patients and parents should be alerted to the possibility of changes in blood glucose control.[43] Tricyclic antidepressants frequently stimulate appetite that can lead to hyperglycemia. Selective serotonin reuptake inhibitors can have appetite-suppressing effects and may also enhance the action of insulin, thereby inducing hypoglycemic episodes.[43,51] Because lithium carbonate seems to have effects that mimic those of insulin as well as stimulate the secretion of glucagon, either hyper- or hypoglycemia may result from its use.[43] Successful treatment of depression may also bring about changes in eating habits, exercise patterns, and the regularity of insulin injections, thereby causing unforeseen changes in blood glucose control.[43]

Anxiety Disorders

Symptoms of anxiety may also be more common in diabetic children and adolescents. As with other diagnoses, anxiety symptoms may occur in the context of poor glycemic control and must be differentiated from hypo- or hyperglycemic conditions. Self-monitoring of blood glucose concentrations can help the patients and parents discriminate between hypoglycemia and anxiety.[43,52] It is often useful to help the child discriminate internalizing symptoms of worry or persistent fears associated with anxiety from physical symptoms of palpitations or diaphoresis associated with a hypoglycemic state. Treatment with antianxiety medications may lead to improved glucose control and even to hypoglycemia.[43,52] Caution is advised when using β-blockers to treat anxiety symptoms, because they can block adrenergic symptoms that are useful in identifying the hypoglycemic state.

Eating Disorders

The coexistence of eating disorders, such as anorexia nervosa and bulimia nervosa, and diabetes has long been recognized in the clinical setting, particularly among female patients. The cause of eating disorders is multifactorial, involving psychological, biologic, genetic, family, social, and environmental factors.[53] Overall, eating disorders that meet DSM-IV diagnostic requirements are more prevalent among adolescents with T1DM than the general population. Subthreshold eating disorder, eating-related disturbances, and misuse of insulin to influence body weight, which pose an increased risk for related medical complications and eating disorders, are common in the female adolescent diabetic population.

Considering the frequency of eating disorders based on DSM-IV criteria, some studies indicate that subjects with diabetes mellitus were 2.4 times more likely to have an eating disorder than controls and 1.9 times more likely to have a subthreshold eating disorder.[54] Smith and colleagues[55] compared adolescent women with diagnoses of scoliosis and IDDM with a normal control group for an increased risk of eating disorders. Of the adolescents with T1DM, 27.5% were found to have either bulimia or binge-eating disorder based on DSM-IV criteria. Although many patients may not meet strict DSM-IV criteria for anorexia nervosa or bulimia, as indicated by refusal to maintain body weight at or above minimally normal weight for age and height and recurrent inappropriate compensatory behavior to prevent weight gain, respectively, deliberate insulin omission was cited as the most common weight loss behavior after dieting. Data suggest that between 15% and 39% of young women with diabetes manipulate their insulin to control their weight, with clinically relevant changes in eating attitudes in boys and girls occurring after their first year of treatment for diabetes.[56] Although some diabetic patients tend to be slightly more overweight than controls, it is the rapid weight gain of rehydration and the anabolic effect of insulin that may be responsible for the rapid weight gain, particularly after diagnosis. Although these changes in eating attitudes were associated with significant changes in body weight, girls were more likely to experience changes in body dissatisfaction, preoccupation with food, body image, and body shape. In relation to bulimia, rather than purging, many diabetic women reduce their dose of insulin to achieve a similar calorie-voiding effect.[57] The availability of this method of weight control, together with dietary restrictions imposed by the diabetes regimen, may explain why many diabetic patients may report less dieting to lose weight, even though they report more binge eating.[54]

Such eating disorders or disturbances in adolescents with T1DM pose a particular health risk in that they are associated with impaired metabolic control and about a 3-fold increase in the risk of diabetic retinopathy.[54] For the clinician, these findings emphasize the importance of considering an eating disorder, or at least disturbed eating, as a cause of poor control of hemoglobin HbA_{1c} control in young women with diabetes.[58]

FAMILY AND DEVELOPMENTAL FACTORS

Consideration of family functioning in families with children with IDDM has a long history. Minuchin and colleagues[59,60] in the 1970s described "psychosomatic" families. These families were described as possibly manifesting 1 of 4 maladaptive transactional patterns: enmeshment, overprotectiveness, rigidity, and lack of conflict resolution. Although the finding has not been clearly replicated, it was found that acutely stressful family interactions could lead to elevated blood glucose levels.

Since Minuchin's original work, there have been many investigations exploring the relationships of family factors mediating treatment adherence, effects of parental mental health issues on disease course, marital difficulties and its effect on the child with diabetes, and developmental aspects of the family and the child with a chronic illness. More recent work is looking at treatment approaches to the family, including multisystemic therapy (MST),[61,62] office-based parent support,[63] and the effect of psychoeducation.[64] This is described in greater detail in the later discussion.

In any chronic illness, an understanding of the psychosocial context of the child's life is critical to managing illness-related behavior and achieving adherence to management regimens that are often painful or uncomfortable and often in conflict with expectable developmental processes. For T1DM, the maintenance of treatment regimens is clearly related to medical outcomes. Short-term consequences of inadequate monitoring of blood glucose, changes in diet or exercise, or problems in insulin administration can potentially lead to seizures, unconsciousness, and death. Poor glycemic control can eventually cause blindness, renal failure, stroke, and myocardial infarction. The seriousness of these outcomes generates a great deal of understandable anxiety in parents and providers, anxiety that often does not yield improvements in treatment adherence, and which may, in fact, lead to conflict, resistance, and additional difficulty.

Understanding family and developmental factors in all pediatric illness and the need for family-based interventions is increasingly being addressed.[65] An understanding of illness-related behaviors in the child or adolescent and of the stress and emotional responses experienced by parents are critical if health care providers are to be effective in achieving helping the patients manage their illnesses effectively. In all serious illnesses in childhood and adolescence, parents can be expected to experience varying degrees of stress and frustration, which may lead to anxiety, depression, alterations in the marital relationship, and difficulties in the relationship with the child. When an illness causes ongoing disability, parents may need to grieve a real loss. These responses in parents are often associated with outcomes in the child, both morbidity (quality of life, psychosocial adjustment, physical complications) and mortality.

Adjustment to the illness and establishment of effective patterns of management of the illness are critical with T1DM. Adherence to treatment regimens and maintenance of metabolic control, while difficult for some to achieve during childhood, often becomes much more difficult with the transition to adolescence.[66] Problematic family interactional factors such as high levels of conflict and low cohesion are associated with poorer adherence to treatment regimens, poorer metabolic control, and worse health outcomes.[67,68]

The Effect of T1DM on Parents and Families

The diagnosis of T1DM in a child or adolescent is often an acute stressor in the lives of parents. They must quickly absorb a substantial amount of new and disturbing information. The physical demands of care are significant, involving blood glucose monitoring, insulin administration, attempts to regulate diet and activity, and time-consuming office visits and calls. Ongoing needs of the ill child's siblings, other family members, and work must be dealt with, and feelings of inadequacy or helplessness are understandable. Many parents experience subthreshold symptoms of distress and mood disturbance after the diagnosis.[40] A significant minority continues, weeks and months later, to experience anxiety and depression.[69] One study observed 22% of mothers of children with T1DM to have clinically significant levels of depression.[70] A study of pediatric parenting stress, as defined by the Pediatric Inventory for Parents, assessing the parents' communication with others, emotional functioning (eg, sleep, mood), the stress of performing the medical regimen, and effects on role functioning (eg, ability to work, care for other children) found that those who experienced a lower sense of self-efficacy in managing the child's medical care and greater parenting stress were more likely to report clinically significant symptoms of anxiety or depression.[71]

The experience of having a child with T1DM is a challenge for the parents' marriage, with consequences for the child's medical and psychosocial outcome. Mothers typically take on most child care, management of the illness, and communication with providers. In the study on parenting stress mentioned earlier, anxiety and depression were greater for mothers than fathers. The presence of each spouse participating in the child's care was a protective factor.[71] Higher levels of mother-reported spousal support have been found to be associated with less conflict with an adolescent with T1DM and with greater adherence to treatment.[70] Single-parent families clearly have greater difficulty with management of the illness than parents living together.[72]

Parents' emotional responses and coping styles interact with those of children and adolescents in a reciprocal or transactional manner. Maternal depression is associated with the quality of life and depressive symptoms in children with T1DM.[73] At the same time, maladaptive emotions and behavior on the part of the child add greatly to the stress on a parent.

Effects of the Child's Age or Developmental Level

Developmental considerations of the child or adolescent with IDDM include the child's age at diagnosis, the complexity of disease management, the ability to consent for treatment, and the trajectory through puberty. In many patients, diabetic control during the critical years of adolescence and early adulthood is determined by control established in late childhood.[74] The challenges to psychological adjustment and family interaction vary with the age or developmental level of the child. The cognitive capacity of the child, stability of attachment to parents, need for autonomy and other developmental needs, and medical issues associated with the patient's age all play a role. As children develop, they should gradually become the primary guardians of personal health and primary partners in medical decision making, assuming responsibility from their parents.[75] Developmentally, this involves a significant range of responsibility for self-care, ultimately resulting in responsibility for appropriate food choices, blood glucose monitoring, knowledge of HbA_{1c}, and appropriate insulin dose adjustment predictions to account the wide array of influencing variables.

It is not unusual for preschoolers to have become very ill and experienced an intense life-threatening condition that initially shapes their perception of what it means to have diabetes. Not surprisingly, this perception is also influenced by parental beliefs, expectations, and ability to effectively communicate with the child. Although the preschoolers have little responsibility in managing their diabetic care, they can begin to communicate subjective perceptions of what it feels to be hyper- or hypoglycemic. The greater risk of hypoglycemic episodes in preschool children often results in anxiety on the part of parents. Needle-related pain and distress may be a particular challenge with younger children, but children's ability and willingness to use needles are not age related.[76] Separation from parents, if hospitalization is necessary, can be a great cause of anxiety.

In latency, the child can begin to develop an understanding of the principles of diabetes, management techniques, and decision making related to considerations of consent. It is clear that "informed consent" has only limited direct application in children and adolescents. Only patients who have appropriate decisional capacity and legal empowerment can give their informed consent to medical care. In all other situations, parents or other surrogates provide "informed permission" for diagnosis and treatment of children with the assent of the child when appropriate. If physicians recognize the importance of assent, they empower children to the extent of their capacity.[75,77]

Assent should include at least the following elements[75]:

1. Helping the child achieve a developmentally appropriate awareness of the nature of his or her condition.
2. Telling each child what he or she can expect with tests and treatment.
3. Making a clinical assessment of the patient's understanding of the situation and the factors influencing how he or she is responding.
4. Soliciting an expression of the patient's willingness to accept the proposed care.

A child's refusal to assent to treatment may represent misunderstandings, fears, and concerns, which if initially respected by the clinician, may provide an opportunity for the exploration of refusal and a strengthening of the therapeutic relationship. Although coercion or force may ultimately be necessary for medical reasons, it should be the last resort, keeping in mind the negative consequences of possible increased aversion to medical procedures.

A developmentally appropriate understanding of the nature of diabetes for childhood assent can often be expressed by latency-age children in simple meaningful terms. Describing "hypos" and "hypers" related to "sugar levels," their direct relation well-being, associated somatic feeling of each condition, and the relationship of food/insulin can usually be understood and expressed by these children. Children need to be helped to have some understanding that the benefit of treatment outweighs the problems of discomfort and inconvenience.

A child's expectation of tests and treatment is usually developed over time, as he or she begins to appreciate the regularity of injections. Appreciation of duration of treatment is more abstract however, and children may reference duration to the number of finger sticks throughout the day, rather than the lifetime.

In addition to simply asking the child to explain in his or her own words, making use of natural play can also indicate understanding of the situation and the factors influencing how he or she is responding. Demonstrations on dolls or asking the child how he or she would advise another boy or girl with diabetes is often perceived as fun and can often yield surprisingly insightful interpretations.

Although there has been little research about children's beliefs and goals or their ability to comanage a serious chronic condition, some studies have revealed that some children possess the knowledge, skill, and maturity to make personal decisions about their health care. It has been found that from around 4 years of age, children start to understand the principles and take responsible moral decisions about managing their diabetes. And yet, other research has indicated that instead of age or ability, experience is the salient factor in a child's intellectual and moral competence.[76,77]

In school-aged children with T1DM, parents still have to take very active responsibility for management.[78] Behaviors that are normal for the developmental stage, such as oppositional interactions, emotional liability, and increasing need for independence, can interfere with management. In addition to the life of the child in the family, challenges also arise with respect to school and peer relationships. The needs to regulate or at least monitor dietary intake and physical activity conflict with the child's need to be active with friends, to participate in sports, and to join activities involving food. A particular difficulty and point of conflict is misbehavior at mealtimes, such as playing with food, talking rather than eating, or refusal to eat, which generates anxiety in the parent who is concerned about the need for consistent intake. Such behavior tends to elicit ineffective, overreactive discipline from parents.[79] Patton and colleagues[80] observed that more parental activity, directing or commanding the child to eat, was associated with less eating as the meal progressed. This was not categorically different from mealtime interactions in healthy controls, but it was associated with poorer glycemic control in children with T1DM. An intervention, using principles similar to those of Parent Management Training,[81] effectively improved mealtime conflict by teaching parents to use short, direct commands that are associated with contingent positive attention.[82]

The transition to adolescence is a time when conflict with the family often increases and adherence to treatment regimens often deteriorates.[83] The same hormones that cause growth spurts in a child can also wreak havoc on his or her efforts to keep blood sugar level under control. As growth hormone increases during the early and middle adolescent years, the body becomes less sensitive to insulin. As a result, high glucose levels are common in late adolescents. When an adolescent reaches his or her full growth, these insulin-inhibiting hormones tend to decrease.[84,85] The increased adolescent physical demands of sports, dance, gymnastics, and many other strenuous activities can also change insulin requirements.

Increased autonomy in the formation of personal identity is an important developmental task of adolescence. This developmental task may be more complicated for adolescents with T1DM because at this time in their lives, metabolic control and treatment adherence often deteriorate and less parental involvement in diabetes care has been associated with poorer diabetes outcomes. Adolescents perceive support from family members primarily in the form of tangible support, such as reminding, helping, and even performing many of the self-management tasks.[86] Parent-child conflict is common and may take the form of parental worry and intrusive behaviors or blaming. Late adolescents often feel that their parents have identified them more in terms of the diabetes than their personality. Misunderstanding of the hormonal changes of development may lead to parental accusations of irresponsible diabetes management. Adolescents are most sensitive to being misunderstood and often either blatantly disregard appropriated diabetes management in response or create factitious blood sugar levels to satisfy the parents.

Issues common in adolescence, including the need for separation and a sense of autonomy; the adolescent's sense of invulnerability and propensity to risk taking; concerns about self-image, sexual identity, and peer group affiliation all complicate relationships with parents and management of the illness. At a time when peers are regarded increasingly as capable of managing certain aspects of their life and enjoy increasingly independent function, the adolescents with T1DM experience continuing vigilance on the part of their parents regarding their dietary intake, physical activity, and consistency with blood glucose monitoring and insulin administration.

Clinical practice consensus guidelines for "Diabetes in adolescence" were developed by the International Society for Pediatric and Adolescent Diabetes and published in 2008.[87] Providers who are sensitive to these issues, hoping to be responsive to the adolescent's need for a degree of mastery and autonomy may attempt a "loose" rather than a "tight" level of control of the illness. Parents and providers often need to be active in monitoring and managing treatment. Although adolescents have greater cognitive capacity and diabetes-related problem-solving skills than younger children, they were found to avoid using such skills in social situations in which they conflicted with acceptance by peers.[88] Active monitoring by parents is associated with better control of the illness.[89] Parents, providers, and adolescents need to find a sustainable balance between monitoring of the treatment regimen and allowing the adolescent to feel increasingly competent and independent.

There are clearly some protective factors. Those with more stable family communication and social support and with more positive self-perceptions experience less stress related to their illness and better glycemic control.[90,91]

INTERVENTIONS

Many children and adolescents have some degree of difficulty in maintaining good glycemic control, and a subset of adolescents has serious problems. These chronically poorly controlled patients are likely to experience multiple risk factors, including other family psychopathology, low levels of parental support and monitoring, irregular contact with care providers, lower socioeconomic status, and minority or single-parent homes.[61,92]

As noted earlier, children and adolescents may experience coexisting psychiatric disorders, such as anxiety, depressive disorders, and eating disorders. Other disorders that are fairly common in children and adolescents and not specifically related to diabetes, such as attention-deficit hyperactivity disorder or learning disabilities, may greatly complicate management. If such comorbid disorders are present, the first priority must be to treat them according to appropriate practice parameters. Family conflict may require family psychotherapy, and treatment of depression, anxiety, or other disorders in parents, either related to the child's diabetes or preexisting, may be indicated. Parents may be reluctant to seek help for themselves when they are preoccupied with a child's illness, but they must be helped to see the need to be functioning well if they are to be helpful to their child and families.

Several interventions, including educational programs, cognitive behavioral therapy, coping-skills training, and family-based interventions, specific to the difficulties experienced by families with a diabetic child have been studied. In a recent article, several interventions from different theoretical perspectives showed promise with respect to psychosocial outcomes and health service use, but without definitive effects on metabolic control.[93] A randomized controlled trial of an educational approach, Parent-Adolescent Teamwork, showed significantly decreased family conflict, but no significant effect on glycemic control.[63] A recent review of family-centered interventions indicated promising results with both family conflict and improved HbA$_{1c}$ levels.[94]

The specific and important issue of needle-related distress has been the subject of successful interventions. Distraction, cognitive behavioral treatment (CBT), and hypnosis have shown promising results. CBT is "well established" for procedure-related pain.[95] Operant learning procedures with positive reinforcement including tokens, tangible rewards, or privileges are considered "probably efficacious," with increased adherence to blood glucose monitoring.[96]

MST is an intensive family-centered treatment modality that was originally developed to treat delinquent adolescents and has been extended to psychiatrically ill children and adolescents.[97] It has been adapted to treat chronically poorly controlled adolescents with T1DM.[98–100] The intensive home-based psychotherapeutic approach includes a wide menu of interventions appropriate to the individual patient and family. Family interventions included parent training regarding monitoring and improving communication. Individual interventions, such as CBT, for a depressed adolescent were used as needed. Treatment included collaboration with schools; involvement of peers, community, and extended family; and problem solving around barriers to keeping medical appointments and communicating with providers. A trend was seen regarding improvement of HbA$_{1c}$ levels, with a decrease of 0.8% in the families completing treatment. Although the mean did not decrease to a level considered acceptable, this degree of improvement is associated with improved medical outcomes. The frequency of blood glucose monitoring increased and the number of hospital admissions for diabetic ketoacidosis decreased.

SUMMARY

In summary, the psychosocial adjustment and behavior of patients with T1DM is critical to their medical outcomes and quality of life, and family support, monitoring, and communication are essential levels of consideration. The illness is a significant and ongoing stressor for parents, and it confounds and complicates many aspects of normal child and adolescent development. Several careful studies have delineated important moderators and mediators of outcomes, and promising interventions have been developed and continue to be studied. Pediatricians, family physicians, nurse practitioners, child and adolescent psychiatrists, and other medical and mental health providers need to understand and address psychosocial adaptation to the illness if they are to improve the outcomes of their patients and their families. Protective factors such as family communication skills, spousal support, and enhancement of positive self-perception should be identified and promoted to minimize short- and long-term complications.

REFERENCES

1. Duncan G, Li S, Zhou X. Prevalence and trends of a metabolic syndrome phenotype among U.S. adolescents, 1999–2000. Diabetes Care 2004;27(10):2438–43.
2. Duncan G. Prevalence of diabetes and impaired fasting glucose levels among US adolescents: National Health and Nutrition Examination Survey, 1999–2002. Arch Pediatr Adolesc Med 2006;160(5):523–8.
3. Nelson R, Bremer A. Insulin resistance and metabolic syndrome in the pediatric population. Metab Syndr Relat Disord 2009. [Epub ahead of print].
4. Hedley A, Ogden C, Johnson C, et al. Prevalence of overweight and obesity among US children, adolescents, and adults, 1999–2002. JAMA 2004;291(23):2847–50.
5. Ogden C, Carroll M, Curtin L, et al. Prevalence of overweight and obesity in the United States, 1999–2004. JAMA 2006;295(13):1549–55.
6. Cohen D. Atypical antipsychotics and new onset diabetes mellitus. An overview of the literature. Pharmacopsychiatry 2004;37(1):1–11.
7. Cohen D, Huinink S. Atypical antipsychotic-induced diabetes mellitus in child and adolescent psychiatry. CNS Drugs 2007;21(12):1035–8.
8. Jerrell J, McIntyre R. Adverse events in children and adolescents treated with antipsychotic medications. Hum Psychopharmacol 2008;23(4):283–90.
9. McIntyre R, Jerrell J. Metabolic and cardiovascular adverse events associated with antipsychotic treatment in children and adolescents. Arch Pediatr Adolesc Med 2008;162(10):929–35.
10. Rosenbauer J, Herzig P, von Kries R, et al. Temporal, seasonal, and geographical incidence patterns of type I diabetes mellitus in children under 5 years of age in Germany. Diabetologia 1999;42(9):1055–9.
11. Bell R, Mayer-Davis E, Beyer J, et al. Diabetes in non-Hispanic white youth: prevalence, incidence, and clinical characteristics: the SEARCH for Diabetes in Youth Study. Diabetes Care 2009;32(Suppl 2):S102–11.
12. Felner E, Klitz W, Ham M, et al. Genetic interaction among three genomic regions creates distinct contributions to early- and late-onset type 1 diabetes mellitus. Pediatr Diabetes 2005;6(4):213–20.
13. Tillil H, Köbberling J. Age-corrected empirical genetic risk estimates for first-degree relatives of IDDM patients. Diabetes 1987;36(1):93–9.
14. Berhe T, Postellon D, Wilson B, et al. Feasibility and safety of insulin pump therapy in children aged 2 to 7 years with type 1 diabetes: a retrospective study. Pediatrics 2006;117(6):2132–7.
15. Nimri R, Weintrob N, Benzaquen H, et al. Insulin pump therapy in youth with type 1 diabetes: a retrospective paired study. Pediatrics 2006;117(6):2126–31.
16. Desrocher M, Rovet J. Neurocognitive correlates of type 1 diabetes mellitus in childhood. Child Neuropsychol 2004;10(1):36–52.
17. Hershey T, Perantie D, Warren S, et al. Frequency and timing of severe hypoglycemia affects spatial memory in children with type 1 diabetes. Diabetes Care 2005;28(10):2372–7.
18. Perantie D, Lim A, Wu J, et al. Effects of prior hypoglycemia and hyperglycemia on cognition in children with type 1 diabetes mellitus. Pediatr Diabetes 2008;9(2):87–95.
19. Perantie D, Wu J, Koller J, et al. Regional brain volume differences associated with hyperglycemia and severe hypoglycemia in youth with type 1 diabetes. Diabetes Care 2007;30(9):2331–7.
20. Hershey T, Perantie D, Wu J, et al. Hippocampal volumes in youth with Type 1 diabetes. Diabetes 2010;59(1):236–41.

21. Rankins D, Wellard R, Cameron F, et al. The impact of acute hypoglycemia on neuropsychological and neurometabolite profiles in children with type 1 diabetes. Diabetes Care 2005;28(11):2771–3.

22. McDonnell C, Northam E, Donath S, et al. Hyperglycemia and externalizing behavior in children with type 1 diabetes. Diabetes Care 2007;30(9):2211–5.

23. Cameron F, Kean M, Wellard R, et al. Insights into the acute cerebral metabolic changes associated with childhood diabetes. Diabet Med 2005;22(5):648–53.

24. Blanz B, Rensch-Riemann B, Fritz-Sigmund D, et al. IDDM is a risk factor for adolescent psychiatric disorders. Diabetes Care 1993;16(12):1579–87.

25. Goldston D, Kelley A, Reboussin D, et al. Suicidal ideation and behavior and noncompliance with the medical regimen among diabetic adolescents. J Am Acad Child Adolesc Psychiatry 1997;36(11):1528–36.

26. Kovacs M, Goldston D, Obrosky D, et al. Psychiatric disorders in youths with IDDM: rates and risk factors. Diabetes Care 1997;20(1):36–44.

27. Garton A, Zubrick S, Silburn S. The Western Australian child health survey: a pilot study. Aust N Z J Psychiatry 1995;29(1):48–57.

28. Costello E. Developments in child psychiatric epidemiology. J Am Acad Child Adolesc Psychiatry 1989;28(6):836–41.

29. Bird H. Epidemiology of childhood disorders in a cross-cultural context. J Child Psychol Psychiatry 1996;37(1):35–49.

30. Northam E, Matthews L, Anderson P, et al. Psychiatric morbidity and health outcome in Type 1 diabetes–perspectives from a prospective longitudinal study. Diabet Med 2005;22(2):152–7.

31. Sawyer M, Arney F, Baghurst P, et al. The mental health of young people in Australia: key findings from the child and adolescent component of the national survey of mental health and well-being. Aust N Z J Psychiatry 2001;35(6):806–14.

32. Garrison M, Katon W, Richardson L. The impact of psychiatric comorbidities on readmissions for diabetes in youth. Diabetes Care 2005;28(9):2150–4.

33. Grey M, Boland E, Yu C, et al. Personal and family factors associated with quality of life in adolescents with diabetes. Diabetes Care 1998;21(6):909–14.

34. Smith M, Mauseth R, Palmer J, et al. Glycosylated hemoglobin and psychological adjustment in adolescents with diabetes. Adolescence 1991;26(101):31–40.

35. Kovacs M, Ho V, Pollock M. Criterion and predictive validity of the diagnosis of adjustment disorder: a prospective study of youths with new-onset insulin-dependent diabetes mellitus. Am J Psychiatry 1995;152(4):523–8.

36. Northam E, Todd S, Cameron F. Interventions to promote optimal health outcomes in children with Type 1 diabetes–are they effective? Diabet Med 2006; 23(2):113–21.

37. Grey M, Cameron M, Lipman T, et al. Psychosocial status of children with diabetes in the first 2 years after diagnosis. Diabetes Care 1995;18(10):1330–6.

38. Kovacs M, Mukerji P, Iyengar S, et al. Psychiatric disorder and metabolic control among youths with IDDM. A longitudinal study. Diabetes Care 1996;19(4):318–23.

39. Northam E, Anderson P, Adler R, et al. Psychosocial and family functioning in children with insulin-dependent diabetes at diagnosis and one year later. J Pediatr Psychol 1996;21(5):699–717.

40. Kovacs M, Feinberg T, Paulauskas S, et al. Initial coping responses and psychosocial characteristics of children with insulin-dependent diabetes mellitus. J Pediatr 1985;106(5):827–34.

41. Kovacs M, Goldston D, Obrosky D, et al. Prevalence and predictors of pervasive noncompliance with medical treatment among youths with insulin-dependent diabetes mellitus. J Am Acad Child Adolesc Psychiatry 1992;31(6):1112–9.

42. Liss D, Waller D, Kennard B, et al. Psychiatric illness and family support in children and adolescents with diabetic ketoacidosis: a controlled study. J Am Acad Child Adolesc Psychiatry 1998;37(5):536–44.
43. Jacobson A. The psychological care of patients with insulin-dependent diabetes mellitus. N Engl J Med 1996;334(19):1249–53.
44. Lustman P, Griffith L, Clouse R, et al. Psychiatric illness in diabetes mellitus. Relationship to symptoms and glucose control. J Nerv Ment Dis 1986;174(12): 736–42.
45. Roy M, Roy A, Affouf M. Depression is a risk factor for poor glycemic control and retinopathy in African-Americans with type 1 diabetes. Psychosom Med 2007; 69(6):537–42.
46. Massengale J. Depression and the adolescent with type 1 diabetes: the covert comorbidity. Issues Ment Health Nurs 2005;26(2):137–48.
47. Kanner S, Hamrin V, Grey M. Depression in adolescents with diabetes. J Child Adolesc Psychiatr Nurs 2003;16(1):15–24.
48. Kaminer Y, Robbins D. Insulin misuse: a review of an overlooked psychiatric problem. Psychosomatics 1989;30(1):19–24.
49. Cassidy E, O'Halloran D, Barry S. Insulin as a substance of misuse in a patient with insulin dependent diabetes mellitus. BMJ 1999;319(7222):1417–8.
50. McEwen B, Magariños A, Reagan L. Studies of hormone action in the hippocampal formation: possible relevance to depression and diabetes. J Psychosom Res 2002;53(4):883–90.
51. Goodnick P, Henry J, Buki V. Treatment of depression in patients with diabetes mellitus. J Clin Psychiatry 1995;56(4):128–36.
52. Cox D, Gonder-Frederick L, Polonsky W, et al. A multicenter evaluation of blood glucose awareness training-II. Diabetes Care 1995;18(4):523–8.
53. Dahan A, McAfee S. A proposed role for the psychiatrist in the treatment of adolescents with type I diabetes. Psychiatr Q 2009;80(2):75–85.
54. Jones J, Lawson M, Daneman D, et al. Eating disorders in adolescent females with and without type 1 diabetes: cross sectional study. BMJ 2000;320(7249):1563–6.
55. Smith F, Latchford G, Hall R, et al. Do chronic medical conditions increase the risk of eating disorder? A cross-sectional investigation of eating pathology in adolescent females with scoliosis and diabetes. J Adolesc Health 2008;42(1):58–63.
56. Antisdel J, Chrisler J. Comparison of eating attitudes and behaviors among adolescent and young women with type 1 diabetes mellitus and phenylketonuria. J Dev Behav Pediatr 2000;21(2):81–6.
57. Steel J, Young R, Lloyd G, et al. Abnormal eating attitudes in young insulin-dependent diabetics. Br J Psychiatry 1989;155:515–21.
58. Fairburn C, Peveler R, Davies B, et al. Eating disorders in young adults with insulin dependent diabetes mellitus: a controlled study. BMJ 1991;303(6793):17–20.
59. Minuchin S, Baker L, Rosman B, et al. A conceptual model of psychosomatic illness in children. Family organization and family therapy. Arch Gen Psychiatry 1975;32(8):1031–8.
60. Minuchin S, Fishman H. The psychosomatic family in child psychiatry. J Am Acad Child Psychiatry 1979;18(1):76–90.
61. Ellis D, Naar-King S, Templin T, et al. Improving health outcomes among youth with poorly controlled type I diabetes: the role of treatment fidelity in a randomized clinical trial of multisystemic therapy. J Fam Psychol 2007;21(3):363–71.
62. Ellis D, Podolski C, Frey M, et al. The role of parental monitoring in adolescent health outcomes: impact on regimen adherence in youth with type 1 diabetes. J Pediatr Psychol 2007;32(8):907–17.

63. Anderson B, Brackett J, Ho J, et al. An office-based intervention to maintain parent-adolescent teamwork in diabetes management. Impact on parent involvement, family conflict, and subsequent glycemic control. Diabetes Care 1999;22(5):713–21.
64. Lochrie A, Wysocki T, Burnett J, et al. Youth and parent education about diabetes complications: health professional survey. Pediatr Diabetes 2009;10(1):59–66.
65. Fiese B. Introduction to the special issue: time for family-based interventions in pediatric psychology? J Pediatr Psychol 2005;30(8):629–30.
66. Johnson S, Tomer A, Cunningham W, et al. Adherence in childhood diabetes: results of a confirmatory factor analysis. Health Psychol 1990;9(4):493–501.
67. Anderson B, Holmbeck G, Iannotti R, et al. Dyadic measures of the parent-child relationship during the transition to adolescence and glycemic control in children with type 1 diabetes. Fam Syst Health 2009;27(2):141–52.
68. Cohen D, Lumley M, Naar-King S, et al. Child behavior problems and family functioning as predictors of adherence and glycemic control in economically disadvantaged children with type 1 diabetes: a prospective study. J Pediatr Psychol 2004;29(3):171–84.
69. Chaney J, Mullins L, Frank R, et al. Transactional patterns of child, mother, and father adjustment in insulin-dependent diabetes mellitus: a prospective study. J Pediatr Psychol 1997;22(2):229–44.
70. Lewandowski A, Drotar D. The relationship between parent-reported social support and adherence to medical treatment in families of adolescents with type 1 diabetes. J Pediatr Psychol 2007;32(4):427–36.
71. Streisand R, Mackey E, Elliot B, et al. Parental anxiety and depression associated with caring for a child newly diagnosed with type 1 diabetes: opportunities for education and counseling. Patient Educ Couns 2008;73(2):333–8.
72. Cameron F, Skinner T, de Beaufort C, et al. Are family factors universally related to metabolic outcomes in adolescents with Type 1 diabetes? Diabet Med 2008;25(4):463–8.
73. Jaser S, Whittemore R, Ambrosino J, et al. Mediators of depressive symptoms in children with type 1 diabetes and their mothers. J Pediatr Psychol 2008;33(5):509–19.
74. Cameron F, Smidts D, Hesketh K, et al. Early detection of emotional and behavioural problems in children with diabetes: the validity of the Child Health Questionnaire as a screening instrument. Diabet Med 2003;20(8):646–50.
75. Bioethics Co. Informed consent, parental permission, and assent in pediatric practice. Pediatrics 1995;95:314–6.
76. Alderson P, Sutcliffe K, Curtis K. Children as partners with adults in their medical care. Arch Dis Child 2006;91(4):300–3.
77. Alderson P, Sutcliffe K, Curtis K. Children's competence to consent to medical treatment. Hastings Cent Rep 2006;36(6):25–34.
78. Palmer D, Berg C, Wiebe D, et al. The role of autonomy and pubertal status in understanding age differences in maternal involvement in diabetes responsibility across adolescence. J Pediatr Psychol 2004;29(1):35–46.
79. Wilson A, DeCourcey W, Freeman K. The impact of managing school-aged children's diabetes: the role of child behavior problems and parental discipline strategies. J Clin Psychol Med Settings 2009;16(3):216–22.
80. Patton S, Piazza-Waggoner C, Modi A, et al. Family functioning at meals relates to adherence in young children with type 1 diabetes. J Paediatr Child Health 2009. [Epub ahead of print].

81. Kazdin A. Parent management training: evidence, outcomes, and issues. J Am Acad Child Adolesc Psychiatry 1997;36(10):1349–56.
82. Stark L, Jelalian E, Powers S, et al. Parent and child mealtime behavior in families of children with cystic fibrosis. J Pediatr 2000;136(2):195–200.
83. Drotar D, Ievers C. Age differences in parent and child responsibilities for management of cystic fibrosis and insulin-dependent diabetes mellitus. J Dev Behav Pediatr 1994;15(4):265–72.
84. Effect of intensive diabetes treatment on the development and progression of long-term complications in adolescents with insulin-dependent diabetes mellitus: Diabetes Control and Complications Trial. Diabetes Control and Complications Trial Research Group. J Pediatr 1994;125:177–88.
85. Amiel S, Sherwin R, Simonson D, et al. Impaired insulin action in puberty. A contributing factor to poor glycemic control in adolescents with diabetes. N Engl J Med 1986;315(4):215–9.
86. Weinger K, O'Donnell K, Ritholz M. Adolescent views of diabetes-related parent conflict and support: a focus group analysis. J Adolesc Health 2001;29(5): 330–6.
87. Court J, Cameron F, Berg-Kelly K, et al. Diabetes in adolescence. Pediatr Diabetes 2008;9(3 Pt 1):255–62.
88. Thomas A, Peterson L, Goldstein D. Problem solving and diabetes regimen adherence by children and adolescents with IDDM in social pressure situations: a reflection of normal development. J Pediatr Psychol 1997;22(4): 541–61.
89. Horton D, Berg C, Butner J, et al. The role of parental monitoring in metabolic control: effect on adherence and externalizing behaviors during adolescence. J Pediatr Psychol 2009;34(9):1008–18.
90. Dashiff C, Hardeman T, McLain R. Parent-adolescent communication and diabetes: an integrative review. J Adv Nurs 2008;62(2):140–62.
91. Malik J, Koot H. Explaining the adjustment of adolescents with type 1 diabetes: role of diabetes-specific and psychosocial factors. Diabetes Care 2009;32(5): 774–9.
92. Ellis D, Yopp J, Templin T, et al. Family mediators and moderators of treatment outcomes among youths with poorly controlled type 1 diabetes: results from a randomized controlled trial. J Pediatr Psychol 2007;32(2):194–205.
93. Couch R, Jetha M, Dryden D, et al. Diabetes education for children with type 1 diabetes mellitus and their families. Evid Rep Technol Assess (Full Rep) 2008;(166): 1–144.
94. McBroom L, Enriquez M. Review of family-centered interventions to enhance the health outcomes of children with type 1 diabetes. Diabetes Educ 2009;35(3): 428–38.
95. Powers S. Empirically supported treatments in pediatric psychology: procedure-related pain. J Pediatr Psychol 1999;24(2):131–45.
96. Lemanek K, Kamps J, Chung N. Empirically supported treatments in pediatric psychology: regimen adherence. J Pediatr Psychol 2001;26(5):253–75.
97. Henggeler S, Rowland M, Randall J, et al. Home-based multisystemic therapy as an alternative to the hospitalization of youths in psychiatric crisis: clinical outcomes. J Am Acad Child Adolesc Psychiatry 1999;38(11):1331–9.
98. Ellis D, Frey M, Naar-King S, et al. The effects of multisystemic therapy on diabetes stress among adolescents with chronically poorly controlled type 1 diabetes: findings from a randomized, controlled trial. Pediatrics 2005;116(6): e826–32.

99. Ellis D, Frey M, Naar-King S, et al. Use of multisystemic therapy to improve regimen adherence among adolescents with type 1 diabetes in chronic poor metabolic control: a randomized controlled trial. Diabetes Care 2005;28(7): 1604–10.
100. Ellis D, Templin T, Naar-King S, et al. Multisystemic therapy for adolescents with poorly controlled type I diabetes: stability of treatment effects in a randomized controlled trial. J Consult Clin Psychol 2007;75(1):168–74.

Mental Health and Quality-of-Life Concerns Related to the Burden of Food Allergy

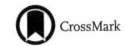

Noga L. Ravid, BA[a], Ronen Arnon Annunziato, PhD[b,c],
Michael A. Ambrose, BA[b], Kelley Chuang, MA[b],
Chloe Mullarkey, BS[b], Scott H. Sicherer, MD[d], Eyal Shemesh, MD[b],
Amanda L. Cox, MD[d,*]

KEYWORDS

• Food allergy • Distress • Bullying • Quality of life

Food allergy seems to be increasing. Based on data from the Centers for Disease Control in the United States, there was an 18% increase in prevalence of food allergy among children from 1997 to 2007, with prevalence estimates currently in the range of 4% to 8%.[1–3] Food allergy differs from other chronic diseases in that affected individuals are in generally good health, but their health may be episodically compromised by acute food-allergic reactions that may be severe or life-threatening. Management of this unpredictable condition may lead to significant distress for food-allergic children and their parents or caregivers. Several studies have examined the effect of food allergy on quality of life (QoL) and emotional impact in children and families, with a particular focus on measures of distress.[4,5] Food allergy has been shown to negatively impact parental, as well as patient, QoL.[5–8] Psychological distress, which includes anxiety, depression, social isolation, and stress, has been demonstrated in children and adolescents with food allergy, although there are variable findings with regard to whether distress is more prevalent among children with food allergy when compared with normative samples.[9]

Several studies have demonstrated a negative impact on health-related QoL, as well as increased distress among food-allergic children and families. However, making comparisons between studies is difficult because of the discrete populations studied, the differing study sizes and geographic locations, and the various methods or tools used to assess psychosocial effects of food allergy on children and their parents.[5] Applying the available findings to a therapeutic end poses an additional challenge in

This article first appeared in Immunol Allergy Clin N Am 2012;32:83–95.
[a] Mount Sinai School of Medicine, New York, NY, USA; [b] Division of Behavioral and Developmental Health, Department of Pediatrics, Mount Sinai Medical Center, 1468 Madison Avenue, New York, NY 10029, USA; [c] Department of Psychology, Fordham University, 441 East Fordham Road, Bronx, NY 10458, USA; [d] Division of Pediatric Allergy and Immunology, Mount Sinai Medical Center, One Gustave L Levy Place, New York, NY 10029, USA
* Corresponding author.
E-mail address: acox@prohealthcare.com

that there is a paucity of literature describing effective interventions. In addition, methods of assessing distress or changes in QoL that result from food allergy vary in the literature. Some studies focus only on parental evaluations,[10,11] while others survey both parents and children.[12] Several studies compared food-allergic children to nonallergic cohorts or to children with other chronic disease, such as diabetes.[13,14] Another study relates subjects' scores to normative scores for the applied tests in the larger population.[15] Moreover, individuals with food allergy often have other atopic conditions that may influence QoL and distress that may be underappreciated in these studies.

The broad range of ages studied should also be taken into consideration. Different developmental stages may influence the divergent manifestations of and means for assessing anxiety in children as opposed to adolescents. Types of questionnaires used and modes of administration also vary, with some studies relying on validated measures and others using modified and nonvalidated tests or qualitative measures such as interviews. Several tools to measure QoL, specifically in food-allergic patients or their families have been introduced and validated only recently.[5,7,8,16]

This article discusses recent information concerning the effects of food allergy on parent and child QoL, as well as distress. It notes the limitations of the available evidence and points out where further study is needed. There is a general movement in medicine toward focusing on QoL as an important outcome measure in health and disease.[17,18] The increasing number of articles about these effects in food allergy is an attestation to the growing importance that the field has started to ascribe to the QoL of affected patients and families.[5] However, our methods of assessment need refinement, especially with regard to the development of evidence-based interventions to improve QoL and reduce distress. Where there is an absence of solid data to back any specific recommendations, the authors provide impressions based on clinical experience with the understanding that, as more data are gathered, our understanding and recommendations will likely need modification.

THE CHILD'S PERSPECTIVE
Studies Examining the Emotional and QoL Consequences of Food Allergy Compared with Other Chronic Illnesses

Assessing the impact of food allergy on QoL requires a point of comparison. Groups evaluated have included children with no food allergy, children with different types or severities of food allergy, children with other allergic disorders, and children with other chronic health conditions. The effects of food allergy on QoL were recently reviewed and summarized.[5] This article offers a critical appraisal of some of the findings to date.

In a study conducted in England, both a self-reporting questionnaire designed by the researchers and an adapted allergy-specific questionnaire were used to survey 20 children with peanut allergy, ages 7 to 12 years, for their fear of adverse outcomes induced by potential or accidental consumption of peanuts.[13] The responses of these children were compared with those of 20 children with insulin-dependent diabetes mellitus. The percentage of children reporting anxiety and the level of anxiety (ranked from high to low) was significantly greater in children with food allergy when compared with children with insulin-dependent diabetes mellitus. In a comparison of food allergy and chronic disease performed in the Netherlands, 98 individuals with various food allergies were surveyed within a larger group of 758, ages 12 to 25 years, with chronic acquired digestive diseases, including inflammatory bowel diseases, chronic liver diseases, congenital disorders, and celiac disease.[14] The survey included a self-reporting questionnaire and the Hospital and Anxiety Depression Scale to probe for burden of disease as measured by leisure activity, sexuality, education, work, and finances. The study found that individuals with food allergy experienced daily disease burden with an impact on school and leisure activities, comparable in several categories to other chronic digestive disorders.

In another study performed in the Netherlands, QoL of food-allergic individuals was compared with that of the general population, as well as to patients with other chronic diseases.[15] Generic QoL questionnaires were completed by food-allergic children (8–12 years), adolescents (13–17 years), and adults (≥18 years). QoL scores were compared with published scores for individuals with irritable bowel syndrome, diabetes mellitus, and rheumatoid arthritis. Food-allergic children and adolescents reported poorer QoL than patients with diabetes mellitus, but had better QoL scores than patients with rheumatoid arthritis, asthma, or irritable bowel syndrome. In addition, food-allergic adolescents and adults showed impairments in QoL compared with the general population. Children, however, demonstrated the least QOL impairment due to food allergy.

Comparisons of these studies are interesting but have limitations due to their differing methodologies and study subjects. Although the findings of Avery and colleagues[13] relate to anxiety while those of Flokstra-de Blok and colleagues[15] relate to QoL, both groups found that food-allergic individuals scored worse than diabetic patients did in these respective psychosocial domains. On the other hand, Calsbeek and colleagues[14] found that comparison of food allergy to a chronic, high somatic-impact disease such as inflammatory bowel disease revealed a lesser social impairment in food allergy. This is consistent with Flokstra-de Blok and colleagues'[15] report of better QoL in food-allergic patients compared with patients with irritable bowel syndrome, asthma, and rheumatoid arthritis. The findings of these studies collectively suggest that the emotional effects seen in patients with food allergy are not easily comparable to those encountered in other disease processes. The clinical manifestations of food allergy are largely episodic in that the disorder is generally not apparent unless or until an allergic reaction occurs. This distinctive characteristic of food allergy may contribute to features of increased anxiety (about the development of acute reactions) but may also result in a lesser impact on socialization when compared with a less episodic, chronic illness such as diabetes. More comparative data are needed before further conclusions can be made.

Studies that Primarily Investigate Children with Food Allergy

Studies comparing food-allergic children to each other, rather than to non–food-allergic cohorts, have suggested additional factors affecting food allergy-related distress and QoL, including epinephrine prescription, history of anaphylaxis, and perception of competence in managing personal health.

In a British study, 41 children (ages 6–16 years) with peanut and tree nut allergies and their mothers completed questionnaires to assess perceived stress and QoL.[12] Children who were not prescribed epinephrine showed greater distress. Distress was not, however, associated with whether or not the child actually carried the prescribed autoinjector. Of note, prior severity of allergic reaction, including anaphylaxis, did not significantly influence child and maternal levels of distress.

Another study, also conducted in England, focused on the impact of awareness and negative-versus-positive perceptions of food allergy on anxiety.[19] Of 162 young adults (ages 15–20 years) who were surveyed at a university, 24 self-reported allergy to certain foods. All completed a Perceived Health Competence Scale and a State-Trait Anxiety Inventory (STAI). As expected, allergic patients were more anxious than those who did not report having allergy. Interestingly, within the small group of

24 food-allergic individuals, those who reported feeling more competent in handling their illness had higher anxiety levels compared with those who reported less competence. Objective assessment of patient levels of "perceived health competence" revealed that most patients who self-reported themselves as "highly competent" did not know the meaning of the term "anaphylaxis." This suggests that self-reported levels of "perceived health competence" in this study were unreliable and unlikely to signify true proficiency in disease management. Nonetheless, the investigators speculated that the association between participants' reported feelings of better competency in managing their illness, as well as increased anxiety, could be attributed to the fact that an increased understanding of food allergy could contribute to a heightened awareness of its risks.[15]

An alternate explanation for the association between anxiety and perceived health competence may be that anxiety prompts patients to inquire more about their illness and thus leads to self-reported higher competence. Based on this conjecture, anxiety among the adolescents surveyed may have contributed to a report of higher competence, rather than competence leading to a report of anxiety, even in cases where patients misjudged or overestimated their knowledge about food allergy. Thus, anxious patients may be more motivated to learn about their disorder, and educating them to become truly competent in managing their food allergy could perhaps decrease their anxiety. On the other hand, as inferred from these findings, patients with food allergy may develop increased anxiety as they learn more about their illness. These seemingly contradictory interpretations would lead to entirely different approaches to patients with food allergy. Accordingly, conclusions derived from cross-sectional studies involving self-reported symptoms or attitudes must be considered cautiously because self-reports do not always faithfully or completely represent the real attitudes, knowledge, or symptoms of the reporting individuals.

Although distress or anxiety are usually perceived as negative emotions that lead to suffering, in fact, some level of anxiety may be adaptive and can lead to better disease management and reduce risk-taking behaviors. Indeed, risk-taking behaviors, such as knowingly ingesting unsafe foods or not carrying prescribed epinephrine, have been noted in adolescents and young adults. In a survey of 13- to 21-year-old food-allergic patients in the United States, alarmingly high rates of risk-taking were reported (ie, 54% reported purposely ingesting unsafe foods and only 61% reported always carrying epinephrine).[20] Those who reported more unsafe behaviors also reported being less concerned about their allergy, and reported feeling "different" more often than those who took fewer risks.

The QoL of children with food allergy and the QoL of their parents has been the focus of several recent studies, as reviewed by Lieberman and Sicherer.[5] QoL of teenagers living with food allergy has been evaluated in the context of developing a specific questionnaire to assess QoL in this group of patients.[7] Teenagers identified limitations on social activities, not being able to eat what others were eating, and limited choice of restaurants as the areas with most adverse impact on their QoL.

Overall, these studies suggest that food-allergic individuals and their families may be more anxious and distressed, and have a lower QoL, when compared with the general population. Increased self-reported "competence" in managing the illness is not necessarily associated with reduced anxiety, although these outcomes may be different if patients cultivate true disease-related competence. Being more anxious, however, is not always problematic, as anxiety can be adaptive and protective against risky behaviors. These findings should be considered when developing therapeutic interventions to improve distress or QoL in patients with food allergy and their families.

THE FAMILY PERSPECTIVE

Awareness of the emotional impact of food allergy has been extended to include the families living with this condition and has led to research on the distress that family members experience and potentially project on one another. The constant fear of anaphylaxis, as well as the consistent vigilance necessary to prevent accidental allergen exposures, can place significant strain on those caring for children with food allergy. Furthermore, parents have the added burden of communicating the risks to others involved in the child's care.

A study of more than 1000 parents of food-allergic children in the United States found overall QoL for caregivers to be variable, although caregivers consistently reported being troubled by social limitations resulting from their child's food allergy.[10] Poor QoL was significantly more likely among caregivers with more knowledge about food allergy and among caregivers whose children had been to the emergency department for food allergy within the preceding year, had multiple food allergies, or were allergic to specific foods (milk, egg, or wheat). In another United States survey of 253 families of food-allergic children, which used a validated, self-administered, children's health questionnaire (CHQ-PF50), parents scored significantly lower (worse) on general health perception, parental emotional impact, and limitation on family activities compared with established norms.[6]

In a study aimed at exploring the challenges faced by parents of young children with food allergy, Rouf and colleagues[21] interviewed a small group of British mothers of food-allergic children and identified themes of parental acclimation to the diagnosis, efforts toward normalizing living with the risks posed by food allergy, and parental concern about their child's identity and inclusion in social life. The study identified that there was a readjustment period to the diagnosis for these mothers that, in different subjects, elicited grief, anxiety, and hope. The study also identified maternal concern over parental responsibility in transferring care of the child to others, teaching others, and cultivating a "normalized" sense of identity in food-allergic children. Another United States study surveyed 2495 parents and found that their children's food allergies adversely affected the parent's personal relationships with the community as well as within the family.[22] Moreover, as reviewed by Klinnert and Robinson,[23] there is concern that parents with extreme levels of anxiety, especially those for whom social interactions with others are also affected, may adopt maladaptive coping strategies. For instance, parents may impose unreasonable social restrictions on the food-allergic child that can interfere with the child's age-appropriate development.

Parental gender may influence the responses and behavioral changes related to food allergy. In one British study of 46 families in which there was a peanut-allergic child, responses of mothers were compared with fathers. Mothers reported greater anxiety and stress than fathers.[24] Importantly, mothers rated the anxiety of their children higher (worse) than the children rated their own anxiety levels. The discrepancy between child and parent reporting of anxiety underscores the importance of directly assessing the child himself or herself for impact of food allergy. This is consistent with the findings of parental reporting of the psychosocial impact of other illnesses on children.[25]

The burden of managing the risks posed to children with food allergy lies with parents or primary caregivers. QoL assessments within families where there is a food-allergic child may show a greater impact on parents than on the children. The influence of a child's food allergy on child and parent QoL were examined in a study comparing QoL for 30 food-allergic children to 15 comparative normal children, as well as QoL between their respective caregivers.[11] The findings indicated that, although food allergy influenced QoL for some children, their parent's QoL was hindered to a greater extent. Furthermore, parents report a better QoL for their food-allergic children than children do when asked directly about themselves, suggesting that direct evaluation of child QoL is necessary.[26]

Comparison of adult and child perspectives on food allergy may reveal specific factors that contribute to child distress from food allergy. LeBovidge and colleagues[9] surveyed 69 children ages 8 to 17 years with food allergy and 141 mothers of food-allergic children ages 2 to 17 years to investigate the influence of maternal anxiety and negative attitudes toward food allergy on the development of child distress using several validated non–disease-specific questionnaires. Scores for anxiety, depression and social stress symptoms in children with food allergy were comparable to average normative child distress scores. The results of this study highlight resilience among children with food allergy. Greater distress was found only in children with a negative approach to food allergy and in younger children of mothers with greater anxiety.

Herbert and Dahlquist[27] examined food allergy as it relates to anxiety, depression, and the impact on autonomy and the influence of parental behavior for 86 food-allergic young adults ages 18 to 22 years. Responses were compared with 344 healthy individuals of the same age. Three nonstandardized questionnaires and several standardized ones were administered. The investigators found that food-allergic participants and healthy participants scored similarly with regard to social self-confidence, autonomy, depression, and anxiety. The subgroup of food-allergic individuals who had a perceived experience of anaphylaxis described greater anxiety about their condition and rated their parents as more overprotective in comparison with food-allergic individuals without a perceived experience of anaphylaxis. The investigators proposed that anaphylaxis in food-allergic patients is a predictor of psychological distress. Conversely, an experience of anaphylaxis may result in reduced distress if individuals are able to manage and master the allergic reaction; thus, the relationship between anaphylaxis and long-term distress requires further investigation.[12]

It is evident from the publications cited above that QoL is negatively affected in families of children who suffer from food allergy. Furthermore, several studies suggest that there is a greater impact on QoL of parents than on the QoL of food-allergic children themselves, at least in the younger age groups. It has not yet been well established whether anxiety is more prevalent among families of children with food allergy than in the general population or compared with families coping with other illnesses. When anxiety is substantially increased, it is likely to be high in both the caretaker and the child. Parental anxiety levels, patient perceptions of food allergy, and coping mechanisms all likely have marked effects on the anxiety and adaptive behaviors of children with food allergy.

The Impact of Oral Food Challenges

Management of pediatric food allergy often involves supervising oral food challenges to either confirm the diagnosis of a food allergy (by positive oral food challenge), or to determine tolerance or resolution of a particular food allergy (by negative oral food challenge). An intervention such as an oral food challenge may result in health-related QoL changes over time for patients and families affected by food allergy.

A few studies have attempted to determine parental anxiety levels related to the performance of oral food challenges.[28–31] Anxiety levels were evaluated in parents of 57 Dutch children with suspected peanut or hazelnut allergy who underwent double-blind placebo-controlled food challenges (DBPCFC) using the Spielberger STAI.[28] Results were compared with Dutch normative values, as well as with parents who refused DBPCFC. The investigators found that parents of children with suspected peanut or hazelnut allergy had high levels of STAI anxiety compared with normal. However, after DBPCFC, state anxiety was significantly lower, regardless of whether their children passed or failed the oral food challenge. Lower state anxiety was maintained even 1 year after food challenge.

In another study, a questionnaire was completed by parents of children with egg allergy. Parents of children who did not undergo food challenge were compared with parents of children who did undergo an open oral food challenge to egg, including 27 who had positive challenges and 57 who had negative challenges to egg. Similar to the above findings among parents of peanut or hazelnut-allergic children, Kemp and colleagues[29] found that performance of an egg oral challenge was associated with reduced adverse parental concerns for most parameters related to expectations about their children's egg allergy, regardless of challenge outcome. These investigators concluded that the experience of an oral food challenge provided parents with greater certainty about their child's food allergy. DunnGalvin and colleagues[30] found comparable results for parental food-allergy QoL using the Food Allergy Quality of Life–Parent Form in a sample of children 0 to 12 years of age undergoing oral food challenges. Scores did improve after oral food challenges for parents of children who had negative challenges, as well as for those whose children had positive challenges.

The studies so far do suggest that oral food challenges may be one area where an intervention may influence or reduce parental anxiety, alleviate distress, and have a positive effect on QoL. However, none of these studies included a random allocation of patients, which precludes any assumption of cause-and-effect relationship between the performance of the food challenge and the apparent association with improved outcomes. It is possible that patients who choose to undergo a food challenge procedure are less anxious then those who do not choose to do it. If so, the difference between anxiety scores in the studied groups could simply reflect a characteristic of those families who tend to proceed with a challenge versus those who do not. The food challenge itself may not be an important factor in relieving anxiety. Although additional research in this area should be conducted before any conclusions or firm recommendations are made, it is possible that, for those who choose to do the challenge, the ensuing information about the child's allergy leads to lesser anxiety. Future studies in this field should be conducted with validated instruments and should assess similar QoL and distress measures among food-allergic children themselves.

FOOD ALLERGY AND BULLYING: AN EMERGING ISSUE

Bullying has devastating effects on children. A study conducted in the United States showed that youth subjected to multiple victimizations experienced more psychological distress and performed worse in school compared with their peers.[32] Another study has shown a clear association between bullying and psychological distress among middle-school boys.[33] In Finland, being bullied in childhood is a predictor of becoming a teenage mother and teen pregnancy has been proposed as one of many long-term outcomes of bullying.[34] School bullying is typically targeted at children that are more vulnerable. A child with food allergy may experience separation from his or her peers during certain social situations, and may have an underlying increased level of anxiety and social stress. These factors may make food-allergic children more susceptible to bullying and its psychological effects.

In a recent study by Lieberman and colleagues,[35] the bullying experience was examined in food-allergic children. A questionnaire designed to assess the nature of teasing, harassment, or bullying of food-allergic patients was distributed to attendees at several regional Food Allergy & Anaphylaxis Network conferences. Most of the surveys were completed by parents of food-allergic children. Of the 353 responses, 24% reported being bullied directly because of food allergy and, of these, most (86%) had experienced multiple episodes of bullying. Most bullying experiences (82%) occurred at school where bullies were mainly classmates. Bullying included teasing or verbal or physical harassment. Of those who experienced bullying, 57% described physical harassment, including being purposely touched with a food allergen. It was also found that 79% of those bullied perceived that they were bullied exclusively because of their food allergy. Furthermore, the respondents cited feelings of sadness, depression, embarrassment, and humiliation because of being bullied; 42.3% felt that the food-allergic child would be harassed or teased again in the future.

Other studies of parent-reported assessment of childhood QoL and anxiety have shown that parents may overestimate child anxiety with respect to food allergy and may not be reliable sources of information regarding their child's experience of food allergy.[24] The findings in the above study on bullying were largely based on parent-completed questionnaires; thus, on parent perception of the food-allergic child's experience. Future studies should directly question the food-allergic child about bullying. Nonetheless, this preliminary study clearly suggests that bullying of food-allergic children does occur and is likely prevalent in the school setting. The extent and correlates of bullying related to food allergy should be further investigated with the aims of raising awareness about this phenomenon and developing interventions to reduce or prevent bullying.

INTERVENTIONS THAT ATTEMPT TO IMPROVE EMOTIONAL OUTCOMES AND QOL

No published studies have evaluated the impact of any intervention on food-allergic children themselves. Studies evaluating the efficacy of educational interventions in other pediatric chronic diseases, including diabetes and asthma, have shown limited improvement in measurable clinical outcomes. For example, in one study of a brief, intensive diabetes educational intervention, patient satisfaction and empowerment improved whereas measures of diabetes such as hemoglobin A1c remained unchanged.[36] Similarly, in a meta-analysis of 37 studies investigating whether asthma self-management education affects children's use of acute care services, emergency department visits and number of hospitalizations decreased, whereas the likelihood of hospitalization and urgent physician visits for asthma remained the same.[37]

To date, only one study has evaluated the impact of an intervention on constructs related to QoL and distress on families who have children with food allergy; however, this study did not use validated measures of those constructs. Lebovidge[38] and colleagues report that a group intervention, consisting of an educational workshop presented to 61 families with food-allergic children, was well accepted. Parents' preintervention and postintervention self-reports indicated increased perception of competence in coping with food allergy and reduced perceived burden of coping with the illness. This study provides preliminary justification for further investigation of group interventions in this population. However, because the study design lacked controls, outcomes were self-reported and not based upon validated instruments, and child-specific assessments were not performed, the authors cannot conclude that the intervention was effective until further studies are performed.

CONCLUSIONS AND FUTURE DIRECTIONS

Box 1 presents a summary of the reviewed articles concerning findings related to QoL, anxiety, and distress in food-allergic patients and their families. Although QoL is invariably reported to be adversely affected, there are discrepancies among reports with

Box 1		
Reviewed articles categorized by construct and outcome		
Construct	**Parents and Family**	**Patients**
QoL	*Decreased*	*Decreased*
	• Lieberman and Sicherer,[5] 2011	• Resnick et al,[7] 2010
	• Gupta et al,[22] 2010	• Flokstra-de Blok et al,[15] 2010
	Variable	
	• Springston et al,[10] 2010	
Anxiety	*Increased*	*Increased*
	• Rouf et al,[21] 2011	• Avery et al,[13] 2003
	• Klinnert et al,[23] 2008	• Calsbeek et al,[14] 2006
	• King et al,[24] 2009	
		No change
		• Lebovidge et al,[9] 2009
		• Herbert and Dahlquist,[27] 2008
Distress	—	*Increased*
		• Cummings et al,[12] 2010

regard to the impact of food allergy on distress and anxiety in children. Some articles demonstrate a clear correlation between the two, although others find no significant association. The use of qualitative as opposed to quantitative methods of study, as well as general as opposed to food allergy-specific instruments, may partially account for the variance in findings. Of note, the sample sizes are generally too small to merit definitive conclusions about the rate or level of distress in food-allergic children compared with children who do not have food allergy. The authors also observe that many of the patient populations recruited for these studies come from backgrounds of high education or income, are already attending an advocacy conference, or are in the care of highly focused allergists. Increasing the diversity of participating subjects with respect to income, health care access, ethnicity, and advocacy awareness will yield more information.

In addition, even when anxiety scales are used, investigators do not use "event-specific" anxiety but rather anxiety traits or states. Those may be less relevant constructs in this population because anxiety in food allergy is frequently related to a specific event, or to a fear about an event, and should be evaluated as such. In addition, the mere demonstration of increased distress in food-allergic children does not imply a pathologic reaction to the illness. Evaluation of correlates of event-specific distress in larger samples, with QoL and other constructs as the outcome variable, would enable an understanding of a threshold of distress in this group of patients. Only beyond that threshold could distress be considered maladaptive. Conversely, levels of distress below that threshold could be desirable. Finally, a total lack of distress may be maladaptive and a cause for concern in the food-allergic population because it could lead to excessive risk-taking.

The experience of being bullied has only recently been studied in the context of food allergy. Additional studies of patients, and potentially of those involved in bullying, are needed to explore the association between bullying and food allergy, as well as whether fear of being bullied contributes to anxiety in children with food allergy. Other considerations might include whether the type and severity of food allergy has an impact on the frequency and form of bullying. Additional research is needed to distinguish between outcomes found via parental reporting versus child reporting of the influence of food allergy on the experiences of being bullied. Of particular interest would be whether parents are aware of most cases of bullying and how bullying is managed when parents are aware.

Parents undoubtedly have a major influence on children's psychological response to their food allergy, and this deserves further exploration. Another unresolved inquiry is whether food allergy and anxiety are organically associated via a genetic link (eg, manifestations of an altered sympathetic nervous system), or whether anxiety develops because of learning patterns, as reviewed recently.[4] Concerning learning patterns, in some patients it may be that increased perceived competency in managing food allergy will lead to increased anxiety.[19] However, it may be that patients who are anxious at baseline are more likely to seek further knowledge about their illness. A cause-and-effect relationship between disease knowledge and distress in food allergy has not yet been substantiated. One pilot study indicated that educational workshops might increase perceived competence in parents.[38] Additional well-designed studies are needed to further examine the outcomes of educational interventions on QoL and distress, as well as to clarify the relationship between knowledge about food allergy and patient or parent anxiety.

SUMMARY

The study of food allergy-related mental health and QoL is truly in its infancy, thus further research is desired in each area reviewed. Based on findings from the available studies in the field, the authors propose the following recommendations with the caveat that, as understanding of the psychosocial impact of food allergy evolves, these recommendations may need to be modified or completely changed.

1. It is important to evaluate event-related anxiety in children with food allergy and their parents as a part of routine clinical visits, because anxiety can affect QoL and illness perception. Both very little and very marked anxiety in either the patient or parent should be of concern.
2. Age-appropriate, validated, food allergy-specific assessments of QoL are available and should be used to evaluate the QoL concerns of food-allergic children and their parents. Food allergy decreases QoL owing to its restrictive effects on diet patterns, social activities, and the need to avoid certain circumstances in which there may be a risk of an accidental exposure to a food.
3. It is not yet clear how to improve QoL in affected patients and families, but several opportunities do exist. To name just a few, a diagnostic test such as a food challenge may improve QoL by confirming persistence versus tolerance of a food allergen, demonstrating appropriate management of an allergic reaction, or reaffirming the extent of avoidance that is needed to protect the patient.[29,30] The provision of more focused information may achieve a similar goal as suggested recently.[39]
4. Some understanding of food allergy is important for patients so that they can manage their illness; however, more knowledge may be associated with increased anxiety and decreased QoL. Thus, it is important to impart knowledge about the illness in a supportive and reassuring way, and to emphasize that successful management of food allergy is possible and, under most circumstances, should not lead to significant disability.

5. Bullying is an emerging concern. Clinicians should inquire about bullying at routine visits.
6. Potentially promising targets for intervention include specific QoL concerns, distress (if excessive), increased knowledge about the illness, and education about coping.
7. Schools are where children socialize most, so a child's safety and comfort in school lunch settings are crucial. In addition, schools are the sites of most bullying in this population.[35] Therefore, the arrangements made by schools to accommodate the child's needs should be of interest to practitioners who may be called on to advocate for a food-allergic child's specific needs.[39,40]
8. When there is a concern about excessive distress or anxiety, allergists and primary care providers should consider referral to a mental health provider or suggest the use of integrated centers that have a psychiatrist or psychologist on staff.

REFERENCES

1. Branum AM, Lukacs SL. Food allergy among children in the United States. Pediatrics 2009;124(6):1549–55.
2. Gupta RS, Springston EE, Warrier MR, et al. The prevalence, severity, and distribution of childhood food allergy in the United States. Pediatrics 2011;128(1): e9–17.
3. Sicherer SH. Epidemiology of food allergy. J Allergy Clin Immunol 2011;127(3): 594–602.
4. Cummings AJ, Knibb RC, King RM, et al. The psychosocial impact of food allergy and food hypersensitivity in children, adolescents and their families: a review. Allergy 2010;65(8):933–45.
5. Lieberman JA, Sicherer SH. Quality of life in food allergy. Curr Opin Allergy Clin Immunol 2011;11(3):236–42.
6. Sicherer SH, Noone SA, Munoz-Furlong A. The impact of childhood food allergy on quality of life. Ann Allergy Asthma Immunol 2001;87(6):461–4.
7. Resnick ES, Pieretti MM, Maloney J, et al. Development of a questionnaire to measure quality of life in adolescents with food allergy: the FAQL-teen. Ann Allergy Asthma Immunol 2010;105(5):364–8.
8. Cohen BL, Noone S, Munoz-Furlong A, et al. Development of a questionnaire to measure quality of life in families with a child with food allergy. J Allergy Clin Immunol 2004;114(5):1159–63.
9. Lebovidge JS, Strauch H, Kalish LA, et al. Assessment of psychological distress among children and adolescents with food allergy. J Allergy Clin Immunol 2009; 124(6):1282–8.
10. Springston EE, Smith B, Shulruff J, et al. Variations in quality of life among caregivers of food allergic children. Ann Allergy Asthma Immunol 2010;105(4):287–94.
11. Valentine AZ, Knibb RC. Exploring quality of life in families of children living with and without a severe food allergy. Appetite 2011;57(2):467–74.
12. Cummings AJ, Knibb RC, Erlewyn-Lajeunesse M, et al. Management of nut allergy influences quality of life and anxiety in children and their mothers. Pediatr Allergy Immunol 2010;21(4 Pt 1):586–94.
13. Avery NJ, King RM, Knight S, et al. Assessment of quality of life in children with peanut allergy. Pediatr Allergy Immunol 2003;14(5):378–82.
14. Calsbeek H, Rijken M, Bekkers MJ, et al. School and leisure activities in adolescents and young adults with chronic digestive disorders: impact of burden of disease. Int J Behav Med 2006;13(2):121–30.

15. Flokstra-de Blok BM, Dubois AE, Vlieg-Boerstra BJ, et al. Health-related quality of life of food allergic patients: comparison with the general population and other diseases. Allergy 2010;65(2):238–44.

16. Flokstra-de Blok BM, DunnGalvin A, Vlieg-Boerstra BJ, et al. Development and validation of a self-administered Food Allergy Quality of Life Questionnaire for children. Clin Exp Allergy 2009;39(1):127–37.

17. Tyedin K, Cumming TB, Bernhardt J. Quality of life: an important outcome measure in a trial of very early mobilisation after stroke. Disabil Rehabil 2010; 32(11):875–84.

18. Ganz PA, Land SR, Geyer CE Jr, et al. Menstrual history and quality-of-life outcomes in women with node-positive breast cancer treated with adjuvant therapy on the NSABP B-30 trial. J Clin Oncol 2011;29(9):1110–6.

19. Lyons AC, Forde EM. Food allergy in young adults: perceptions and psychological effects. J Health Psychol 2004;9(4):497–504.

20. Sampson MA, Munoz-Furlong A, Sicherer SH. Risk-taking and coping strategies of adolescents and young adults with food allergy. J Allergy Clin Immunol 2006; 117(6):1440–5.

21. Rouf K, White L, Evans K. A qualitative investigation into the maternal experience of having a young child with severe food allergy. Clin Child Psychol Psychiatry 2011. [Epub ahead of print].

22. Gupta RS, Springston EE, Smith B, et al. Food allergy knowledge, attitudes, and beliefs of parents with food-allergic children in the United States. Pediatr Allergy Immunol 2010;21(6):927–34.

23. Klinnert MD, Robinson JL. Addressing the psychological needs of families of food-allergic children. Curr Allergy Asthma Rep 2008;8(3):195–200.

24. King RM, Knibb RC, Hourihane JO. Impact of peanut allergy on quality of life, stress and anxiety in the family. Allergy 2009;64(3):461–8.

25. Shemesh E, Newcorn JH, Rockmore L, et al. Comparison of parent and child reports of emotional trauma symptoms in pediatric outpatient settings. Pediatrics 2005;115(5):e582–9.

26. van der Velde JL, Flokstra-de Blok BM, Dunngalvin A, et al. Parents report better health-related quality of life for their food-allergic children than children themselves. Clin Exp Allergy 2011;41(10):1431–9.

27. Herbert LJ, Dahlquist LM. Perceived history of anaphylaxis and parental overprotection, autonomy, anxiety, and depression in food allergic young adults. J Clin Psychol Med Settings 2008;15(4):261–9.

28. Zijlstra WT, Flinterman AE, Soeters L, et al. Parental anxiety before and after food challenges in children with suspected peanut and hazelnut allergy. Pediatr Allergy Immunol 2010;21(2 Pt 2):e439–45.

29. Kemp AS, Allen CW, Campbell DE. Parental perceptions in egg allergy: does egg challenge make a difference? Pediatr Allergy Immunol 2009;20(7):648–53.

30. DunnGalvin A, Cullinane C, Daly DA, et al. Longitudinal validity and responsiveness of the Food Allergy Quality of Life Questionnaire–Parent Form in children 0-12 years following positive and negative food challenges. Clin Exp Allergy 2010;40(3):476–85.

31. Strinnholm A, Brulin C, Lindh V. Experiences of double-blind, placebo-controlled food challenges (DBPCFC): a qualitative analysis of mothers' experiences. J Child Health Care 2010;14(2):179–88, 32.

32. Holt MK, Finkelhor D, Kantor GK. Multiple victimization experiences of urban elementary school students: associations with psychosocial functioning and academic performance. Child Abuse Negl 2007;31(5):503–15.

33. Dao TK, Kerbs JJ, Rollin SA, et al. The association between bullying dynamics and psychological distress. J Adolesc Health 2006;39(2):277–82.

34. Lehti V, Sourander A, Klomek A, et al. Childhood bullying as a predictor for becoming a teenage mother in Finland. Eur Child Adolesc Psychiatry 2011; 20(1):49–55.

35. Lieberman JA, Weiss C, Furlong TJ, et al. Bullying among pediatric patients with food allergy. Ann Allergy Asthma Immunol 2010;105(4):282–6.

36. George JT, Valdovinos AP, Russell I, et al. Clinical effectiveness of a brief educational intervention in Type 1 diabetes: results from the BITES (Brief Intervention in Type 1 diabetes, Education for Self-efficacy) trial. Diabet Med 2008;25(12): 1447–53.

37. Coffman JM, Cabana MD, Halpin HA, et al. Effects of asthma education on children's use of acute care services: a meta-analysis. Pediatrics 2008;121(3): 575–86.

38. LeBovidge JS, Timmons K, Rich C, et al. Evaluation of a group intervention for children with food allergy and their parents. Ann Allergy Asthma Immunol 2008; 101(2):160–5.

39. Sicherer SH, Mahr T. American Academy of Pediatrics Section on Allergy and Immunology. Management of food allergy in the school setting. Pediatrics 2010;126(6):1232–9.

40. Young MC, Munoz-Furlong A, Sicherer SH. Management of food allergies in schools: a perspective for allergists. J Allergy Clin Immunol 2009;124(2): 175–82, 182.e1–4 [quiz: 183–4].

Cognitive Functioning, Mental Health, and Quality of Life in ICU Survivors: An Overview

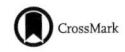

James C. Jackson, PsyD[a,b,*], Nathaniel Mitchell, PhD[c],
Ramona O. Hopkins, PhD[d,e,f]

KEYWORDS

- Cognitive impairments • Critical illness • Critical care outcomes
- Psychiatric disorders • Quality of life

There has been increasing awareness of the fact that diseases, treatments, and events (such as surgery or the experience of critical care) often have significant and persistent consequences for cognitive and psychological functioning.[1] Progress in critical care has led to decreased mortality rates among individuals admitted to intensive care units (ICUs). However, for many survivors of critical illness, ICU hospitalization can lead to a life of significant limitations and obstacles, especially with regard to cognitive functioning. Although neurologic dysfunction is not as well studied in the critical care literature as it ought to be, current data suggest a high prevalence of neurologic disturbances in patients with critical illness admitted to medical/surgical (non-neurologic) ICUs.[2–4] Such disturbances can be severe and include encephalopathy and cognitive and psychiatric impairments. Important neurologic disturbances that are common during and after critical care are delirium and long-term cognitive impairments. Emerging research indicates that although these disorders are distinct, they are inextricably linked in critical care. **Fig. 1** shows possible relationships between premorbid state, critical illness, and outcomes. Recent investigations show that delirium is widely prevalent during critical illness and places patients at greater risk for development of

This article first appeared in Anesthesiology Clin 2011;29:751–64.
A version of this article appeared in the 25:3 issue of *Critical Care Clinics*.
[a] Center for Health Services Research, Vanderbilt University Medical Center, Vanderbilt University School of Medicine, 6th Floor MCE Suite 6100, Nashville, TN 37232, USA; [b] VA-Tennessee Valley Health System (VA-TVHS), Alvin C. York (Murfreesboro) Campus, 3400 Lebanon Pike, Murfreesboro, TN 37129, USA; [c] Department of Psychology, Spalding University, 845 South Third Street, Louisville, KY 40203, USA; [d] Department of Psychology, Brigham Young University, Provo, UT 84602, USA; [e] Neuroscience Center, Brigham Young University, Provo, UT 84602, USA; [f] Department of Medicine, Pulmonary and Critical Care Division, Intermountain Medical Center, Murray, UT, USA
* Corresponding author.
E-mail address: james.c.jackson@vanderbilt.edu

Psychiatr Clin N Am 38 (2015) 91–104
http://dx.doi.org/10.1016/j.psc.2014.11.002
0193-953X/15/$ – see front matter © 2015 Elsevier Inc. All rights reserved.

psych.theclinics.com

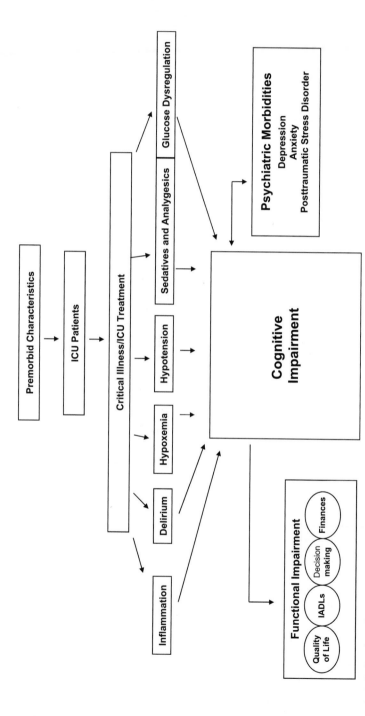

Fig. 1. Relationships between critical illness and outcomes.

cognitive impairment.[5] Further, long-term cognitive impairments may occur in more than half of all ICU survivors and are associated with poor functional outcomes.

DELIRIUM OR ACUTE COGNITIVE OUTCOMES IN ICU PATIENTS

Delirium is a neurobehavioral condition that occurs in a wide variety of health care settings, is associated with adverse outcomes, including death, and is the most common manifestation of acute brain dysfunction during critical illness.[6–8] It is a potentially toxic neuropsychiatric syndrome, characterized by a fluctuating course and pronounced inattention. It is highly prevalent among the hospitalized elderly, affecting between 15% and 20% of hospitalized medical patients,[9] 25% to 65% of surgical patients,[10,11] and as many as 80% of patients in ICU settings.[12] Although delirium was once considered benign, recent evidence has linked it with a variety of adverse outcomes, including prolonged hospitalization, poor surgical recovery, and increased morbidity and mortality.[13–16] Some researchers speculate that delirium may be a marker of subclinical dementia or cognitive impairment that might not otherwise develop for years or decades; indeed, data suggest that common pathogenic mechanisms might underlie development of cognitive impairments in delirium and dementia.[17]

Delirium is linked to poor cognitive outcomes in a variety of patient populations. A review by Maclullich and colleagues,[18] which looked at nine studies published after 2004 on the association between delirium and cognitive decline, documented a strong relationship between these two conditions. Their conclusions echoed those of Jackson and colleagues[19] in the 2004 review on the same topic, which focused on another nine investigations conducted since 2004. Together, these reviews represented a total of 18 investigations—most of them prospective cohort studies—from 1989 to 2008, with a combined total of nearly 4000 patients. These investigations almost uniformly demonstrated, with varying degrees of rigor and sophistication, that the emergence of delirium was a harbinger for greater, more severe, and more persistent neuropsychological decline. Although relevant research to date has focused on the link between delirium and global cognitive impairment, there is emerging evidence to suggest that delirium may be characterized by distinct anatomic patterns and processes.[20] Recent investigations employing sophisticated neuroimaging technologies have demonstrated that delirium results in significant cerebral hypoperfusion in several brain regions, including frontal, temporal, and subcortical regions.[21] Subcortical structures, which appear to mediate key elements of executive functioning, are particularly susceptible to even slight alterations in blood flow because of the small perforating vessels feeding these structures.[22] Evidence from clinical investigations suggests that executive dysfunction commonly develops secondary to reduced blood flow to vulnerable subcortical structures implicated in frontal-subcortical circuitry, even in the absence of frank ischemic injury.[23]

A variety of central nervous system insults, such as stroke and traumatic brain injury, can cause delirium and cognitive impairments, suggesting that widely distributed central nervous system abnormalities likely occur.[24] Neuroimaging data are lacking in critically ill patients with delirium or long-term cognitive impairments. One study found that neuropathologic abnormalities, including significant ventricular enlargement and generalized atrophy, occurred in elderly delirious patients compared with controls.[25] Focal lesions (infarcts and hemorrhage) were observed in frontal and parietal regions in these delirious patients.[25] A study of critically ill patients who underwent CT brain imaging for diminished level of consciousness, confusion, altered mental status, or prolonged delirium found that 61% had abnormalities on brain imaging, including generalized brain atrophy, ventricular enlargement, white matter lesions/hyperintensities, and cortical and subcortical lesions.[26] Although data are limited, future studies using increasingly sophisticated, hypothesis-driven brain imaging techniques will help advance the understanding of the neurologic effects of delirium, its relationship to cognitive impairments after critical illness, and its treatment, while potentially elucidating neuroscientific mechanisms that are now unknown.

PREVALENCE OF COGNITIVE IMPAIRMENT IN ICU SURVIVORS

The terms *cognitive dysfunction* and *cognitive impairment* are often used synonymously, although *impairment* implies a greater degree of permanence in contrast to *dysfunction*, which refers to an acute condition that may change or improve. Recognizing this distinction, it is perhaps most appropriate to discuss ICU survivors in the context of cognitive impairment, because the neuropsychological deficits that characterize these individuals may improve with time, but tend to be permanent in most cases.[27] Among mechanically ventilated general medical ICU survivors, approximately a third or more demonstrate moderate to severe cognitive impairment 6 months after discharge.[28] Among cohorts composed of both medical and surgical ICU survivors, including those with specific conditions such as sepsis and acute respiratory distress syndrome (ARDS), rates of impairment vary widely in part because of assessment timing and methods.[2,4] Among specific populations, notably patients with ARDS, the prevalence of cognitive impairments is particularly high and persistent, with 46% of patients at 1 year[29] and 25% of patients at 6 years reporting ongoing difficulties.[30] Although highly prevalent, cognitive impairment demonstrated by ICU survivors is also often quite severe. For example, the aforementioned ARDS patients with cognitive sequelae all fell below the sixth percentile of the normal distribution of cognitive functioning, displaying marked neuropsychological deficits in wide-ranging areas, including on tasks requiring memory, executive functioning, and mental processing abilities. Impairment does not impact all domains equally, and deficits in some areas rebound more completely than others.

Significant questions exist related to the relationship between premorbid cognitive functioning and the development of subsequent cognitive impairment among ICU survivors.[27] Although many individuals are cognitively normal before the onset of hospitalization, others, particularly those with multiple medical comorbidities that may impact cognition, such as vascular disease, diabetes, chronic obstructive pulmonary disease, and HIV, may have preexisting cognitive impairments.[31,32] They may be particularly vulnerable to the neurologic effects of critical illness. One of the most provocative issues in this regard is whether individuals with preexisting forms of cognitive impairment, particularly conditions such as mild cognitive impairment (MCI) or Alzheimer disease, which are characterized by a natural history of decline, may worsen more rapidly than they otherwise would after neurologic insults such as those occurring during the ICU stay. Conditions such as Alzheimer disease and its common precursor, MCI, affect large numbers of elderly patients—individuals who increasingly undergo and survive intensive care treatment and major surgery and who may be at particular risk to experience potentially toxic syndromes such as delirium.

PERSISTENCE OF COGNITIVE IMPAIRMENTS

It seems that many ICU survivors experience some or marked improvement in cognitive functioning in the year after hospital discharge (those already in the process of cognitive decline at the time of their critical illness may improve relative to their levels of cognitive functioning at hospital discharge, only to return to a pattern of gradual or accelerated deterioration).[4] However, despite demonstrating a clear trajectory of improvement, many individuals continue to have persistent cognitive impairment with time, infrequently returning to their pre-ICU baseline levels. For example 70% of ARDS survivors had cognitive impairments at hospital discharge, but 45% had cognitive impairments at 1 year. There was no improvement in the cognitive impairment rate from 1 to 2 years.[33] A retrospective cohort study of 46 ARDS survivors found 25% had cognitive impairments 6 years after ICU treatment; only 21 patients returned to full-time employment, and all patients with cognitive impairments were disabled.[30] A second study in 30 ARDS survivors had impaired memory, attention, concentration, executive dysfunction, and motor impairments when assessed from 1 to more than 6 years post-hospital discharge (mean 6.2 years).[34] These studies suggest that the cognitive impairments in ARDS survivors are persistent, affect employment, and for a subset of the ICU population are resistant to significant improvement.

It may be that the effects of ARDS on cognitive functioning are accelerated among patients with specific sorts of vulnerabilities, such as frail elderly, although this proposition has largely been unstudied among critically ill patients. Nevertheless, the idea that the effects of ARDS on cognitive function may be magnified among some individuals, such as geriatric patients with preexisting MCI or dementia, is compelling. Although data are lacking, it may be that some ICU survivors suffer from a clinically distinct condition that is referred to as "ICU accelerated dementia." The phenomenon in which the rate of cognitive impairment increases after medical illness has been observed among other populations, including most notably in the well-known neuro-epidemiologic investigation, the Cache County study, which studied progression of dementia in medically ill patients with early Alzheimer disease.[35]

MECHANISMS OF COGNITIVE IMPAIRMENTS

It has been widely recognized that the brain is an immunologically active organ and therefore is vulnerable to systemic inflammatory reactions such as those resulting from sepsis or septic shock, similar to the findings in severe systemic illness. The inflammatory responses are mediated by cytokines, nonantibody proteins that penetrate the blood-brain barrier directly or indirectly to modulate and influence brain activity and potentially alter neurotransmitter release. Studies have shown that increased levels of biologic markers of inflammation, including IL-6 and TNF-α, predict the development of cognitive impairments among older patients without acute illness.[36,37] However, as is true with most cognitive impairments, including the family of dementias, there is probably not a single uniform cause; instead, a number of more or less significant factors interact dynamically with premorbid and genetic variables, resulting in adverse outcomes. Mechanisms of cognitive impairment implicated in the development of brain injury among ICU survivors include hypoxemia,[29] hyperglycemia,[38] delirium duration,[5] and hypotension.[39]

The use of sedatives or analgesics is associated with poor cognitive outcomes in other populations,[40,41] although their role in the development of cognitive impairment after critical illness has been largely unstudied. However, they may be powerfully implicated in the relationship that has been demonstrated between delirium and the emergence of subsequent neuropsychological deficits.[5] That is, sedatives and analgesics, particularly benzodiazepines, contribute to the development of delirium, which in turn is associated with an increased risk for cognitive impairment. Although the specific nature of the relationship between sedatives or analgesics has yet to be fully studied in ICU cohorts and is yet to be elucidated, there are reasons to believe that certain medications or medication classes could contribute to adverse cognitive outcomes, particularly in vulnerable populations. For example, in a recent investigation by

Pomara and colleagues,[42] healthy elderly subjects with the *APOE4* allele, a well-known genetic risk factor for Alzheimer disease, experienced more pronounced cognitive impairment and were slower to recover after acute oral challenge with lorazepam. The cognitive impairment experienced by these subjects was not the result of pharmacokinetic factors, raising the possibility that factors unique to the effects of *APOE4* may have resulted in pronounced vulnerability to drug-related cognitive toxicity. Although the idea that certain genetic alleles may mediate and amplify the effects of specific drugs on the development of cognitive impairment is controversial and not unanimously supported by the literature, it highlights yet another possible mechanism through which neuropsychological deficits in ICU survivors might develop.

DEPRESSION AND ANXIETY IN ICU SURVIVORS

Psychological morbidity, such as depression and anxiety, occurs frequently after critical illness.[43,44] Depression occurs in 25%[33] to more than 50% of survivors of critical illness.[45] Angus and colleagues[45] reported that 50% of ARDS survivors had depression 1 year after treatment, whereas Cheung and colleagues[46] reported a 58% incidence of depression 2 years after ICU discharge. A study of 13 ICUs in four hospitals found that 26% of patients had symptoms of depression 6 months after acute lung injury.[47] Similar rates of depression are reported in 22% to 33% of medical inpatients[48] and in 25% to 28% of patients with cardiac and pulmonary disorders.[49,50] Psychiatric disorders after critical illness may be because of a psychological reaction to the emotional and physiologic stress, sequelae of brain injury sustained as a result of critical illness and its treatment, or both. Medications, physiologic changes, pain, altered sensory inputs, and an unfamiliar environment are all potential contributors in the development of psychological sequelae.[51]

There is little data available about risk factors for depression in survivors of critical illness. Depression is positively associated with longer ICU lengths of stay, longer duration of mechanical ventilation, and greater number of days on sedatives.[52] Two additional studies support the relationship between longer ICU lengths of stay and depression.[43] No information is available regarding factors related to longer ICU lengths of stay that lead to the development of depression. That is, it is not known if it is the time or the longer exposure to other factors such as sedatives or glucose dysregulation that results in depression. For example, a recent study found that hypoglycemia during ICU treatment was associated with greater symptoms of depression 3 months after acute lung injury.[47] Other factors related to depression are higher body mass index, premorbid depression or anxiety, and mean ICU benzodiazepine dose.[47] A study in 13 ICUs from four hospitals found depression at 6 months was related to surgical but not medical or trauma ICU admission, maximum organ failure score, and mean benzodiazepine dose.[53]

Although the above studies are starting to assess relationships between critical illness and ICU treatment with development of depression, research is in its infancy; additional studies are needed to determine risk factors, mechanisms, and potential treatments. Daily sedative interruption did not reduce the prevalence of depression at hospital discharge, but did reduce the rate of depression at 1 year.[54] A study that assessed prevalence of antidepressant treatment found that 37% of ARDS patients were taking antidepressant medications 2 months after ICU discharge.[44] Little is known regarding whether treatment of depression with antidepressant medications improves outcomes.

There is limited information on generalized or nonspecific anxiety in critically ill populations. The prevalence of nonspecific anxiety is less frequently reported than depression, but the rate of anxiety ranges from 23% to 41%.[43,54] The rates of anxiety in ICU survivors is higher than that observed in medical inpatients (5%–20%),[55] but similar to the reported rates of 10% to 40% observed in patients with pulmonary disorders.[56] Potential mechanisms of depression and anxiety in ICU survivors include organ dysfunction, medications, pain,[52] sleep deprivation, ICU treatment, elevated cytokines,[57] stress-related activation of the hypothalamic-pituitary axis, hypoxemia, and neurotransmitter dysfunction due to brain injury. The most frequently identified anxiety disorder is posttraumatic stress disorder (post traumatic stress disorder [PTSD], see discussion in the next section). The prevalence of psychological morbidity is high and research is in its early stages. Future investigations should assess mechanisms, risk factors, and possible interventions.

POST TRAUMATIC STRESS DISORDER IN ICU SURVIVORS

PTSD was once believed to result primarily from experiences such as combat, assault, and exposure to a natural disaster. Experts have recognized that a somewhat broader array of events may indeed be traumatic to individuals, including life-threatening illnesses and surgical procedures. A significant literature has emerged in this regard, particularly as it relates to the development of PTSD after the diagnosis of cancer. Researchers and clinicians are focusing on another experience believed to contribute to PTSD and PTSD symptoms—critical illness and the events associated with ICU hospitalization—although a debate on the prevalence and severity of PTSD in ICU survivors is ongoing.[58]

Of particular interest for ICU clinicians and research is the role of memory in mediating the development of PTSD, because a key impetus for employing strategies to keep critically ill patients heavily sedated has been the concern that memories of their ICU experience could facilitate the development of PTSD.[59] The importance of specific *explicit memories* (memories pertaining to facts and events, which are accessible to consciousness)[24,25] in the generation and maintenance of PTSD is difficult to estimate because they are the basis for nightmares, flashbacks, and intrusive thoughts, and they contribute to avoidant and reexperiencing symptoms. Although a detailed treatment of these issues is beyond the scope of this review, the authors briefly discuss several key findings from the literature as they relate to ICU populations. The preponderance of evidence suggests that the absence of episodic memory for a traumatic event is protective against the development of PTSD; most studies have shown that the risk of PTSD is markedly lower in individuals unable to recall a traumatic event than in those with explicit memory for the event(s).[26,60–63] The literature is not unanimous and is quite narrow in scope, with virtually all relevant studies having been conducted on victims of motor vehicle accidents or other traumas with concomitant traumatic brain injury.[64] Theories of information processing suggest that traumatic memories can be encoded *implicitly* during periods of impaired consciousness and may provide the basis for the generation of PTSD symptoms even if patients are not consciously aware of the memories.[65–68] Also, during periods of impaired consciousness, the encoding of emotional experiences such as panic or severe pain appears to be sufficient for the generation of PTSD symptoms.[69]

Many ICU patients report little, if any, conscious awareness of their critical illness, although as Jones and colleagues[70] have reported, delusional memories, often having violent and paranoid themes, are pervasive among these individuals. Among patients with delirium, particularly hyperactive delirium, psychotic symptoms including visual hallucinations are particularly common.[71,72] These hallucinations and delusions can be extremely gripping and are often characterized by paranoid and traumatic themes involving physical or sexual assault or torture. As is frequently the case, these hallucinations are integrated by patients into a narrative that sometimes involves benign actual events and, as such, tend to be entrenched. Even after hallucinations dissipate, their effects may persist in the form of delusional memories, particularly for those patients who remain convinced that the aversive experiences they remember actually happened. Importantly, sedative medications may be one factor that mediates the development of delusional memories.[73] Delusional memories may exist in the absence of factual memories, and factual memories provide markers of reality and may serve to orient the patient. For example, in one study, daily sedative interruption was associated with fewer symptoms of PTSD,[54] suggesting that even limited factual memories from brief awakening may reduce PTSD. In addition, delusional memories tend to be stable with time and are significantly more persistent than factual memories.[74] Delusional memories may be more refractory to the normal cognitive processes of habituation and reappraisal because they are not well integrated into the long-term memory. Although research is limited, the presence of delusional memories of the ICU is associated with increased levels of anxiety and PTSD.[75,76]

QUALITY OF LIFE IN ICU SURVIVORS

Health-related quality of life has emerged as an important measure of outcome in a variety of disease states and may be particularly important after ICU treatment, where interventions can maintain life but may lead to significant morbidity. Although definitions differ slightly across disciplines, health-related quality of life is defined as a set of causally linked dimensions of health, with biologic/physiologic, mental, physical, social function, cognitive, and health perceptions.[44] Critically ill patients with severe sepsis[77] and prolonged mechanical ventilation[78] have significantly lower quality of life. The quality-of-life scores for ARDS survivors are very low at extubation and then increase substantially at 3 months, with only slight additional improvement by 1 year.[44] The reduced quality of life occurs primarily in physical domains (eg, physical functioning, bodily pain, and role physical)[44] and is associated with pulmonary symptoms,[44] abnormal pulmonary function,[79] and persistent muscle wasting and weakness.[80] The perturbations in quality of life appear to be profound as Rothenhäusler and colleagues[30] state: "…the success of intensive care management of severe diseases such as ARDS is no longer judged solely by its effects on survival but by its influence on patients' psychosocial well-being."

Dowdy and colleagues,[81] in a recent meta-analysis of health-related quality of life in ARDS survivors, found that ARDS survivors consistently had lower quality-of-life scores compared with matched, normative controls at all time points after ICU discharge (from hospital discharge up to 66 months later). The magnitude of the quality-of-life differences between critically ill patients and healthy controls represent a moderate decline in physical domains and mild-to-moderate decline in emotional domains, particularly early after ICU discharge. Improvements in quality of life are uneven and are time- and domain-specific.[33] The greatest gains occur in physical functioning, social functioning, and role physical in the first 6 months, with only modest additional improvements thereafter. Role physical is the singular domain where improvement continues throughout the first several years.[33] Although quality-of-life scores improve with time in most longitudinal studies, these improvements do not necessarily reflect clinical meaningful changes in function. As Herridge and colleagues[80] state, health-related quality of life "will be profoundly influenced by the patient's prior health status and her expectations for a return to premorbid functional status."

The timing of quality-of-life assessment may influence the findings either by exaggerating or by underestimating patient perception of their quality of life relative to their critical illness and ICU treatment. Survivors may have shifting perceptions of their illness and recovery, leading to different responses with time, without a similar objective change in their actual capabilities. Conversely, report improvements in quality of life might be more relevant than objective changes in capabilities in predicting willingness and ability to contribute to society. The influence of the "ICU experience," such as invasive procedures and the amount and quality of caregiver support, on health-related quality of life scores has not been assessed. Given the importance of quality of life as a measure of global outcome in survivors of critical illness, it is imperative that clinicians understand that brain function, musculoskeletal function, and other components of medical care that influence quality of life should also be assessed.

Neurocognitive impairments are a major determinant of the ability to return to work, work productivity, life satisfaction, and reduced quality of life.[82] Two studies found that ARDS patients with cognitive impairment had lower quality of life compared with patients without cognitive impairment.[82] Rothenhäusler and colleagues[30] found that ARDS patients with and without neurocognitive impairments had lower quality of life compared with age- and gender-matched healthy controls. Alternatively, decreased quality of life was not associated with neurocognitive impairments in ARDS survivors or with executive dysfunction in a critically ill medical population.[83] Depression and anxiety are also associated with decreased quality of life for all domains, except physical functioning.[39] A study in patients with acute lung injury found that depression and psychosocial symptoms were associated with lower life satisfaction, but not with physical problems or limitations.[44] Depression correlated with poor functional status and decreased ability to perform activities of daily living in patients with chronic obstructive pulmonary disease.[84] Decreased quality of life on the psychosocial domains (eg, role emotional, mental health, and vitality) is associated with PTSD in ARDS patients.[43] Greater PTSD symptoms are associated with reduced quality-of-life scores.[85] Psychiatric disorders and their relationships with decreased quality of life are undoubtedly multifactorial. Data to date indicate that cognitive and emotional functions are associated with lower quality of life after critical illness. The effects of critical illness and ICU therapies extend well beyond hospital discharge and often lead to significant neurocognitive and psychiatric morbidities and reduced quality of life in survivors.[33,80] The observed morbidities and their adverse impact on quality of life raise questions regarding possible interventions to improve outcomes in these patients.

SUMMARY

The significant and sometimes permanent effects of critical illness on wide-ranging aspects of functioning are increasingly recognized. Among the areas affected are acute and long-term cognitive functioning, depression, anxiety, PTSD, and quality of life. These and other areas are increasingly being studied and indeed are increasingly the focus of clinical attention and investigations. These conditions have been a focus of attention for more than a dozen years, with much improvement occurring in the ability to characterize these phenomena. For instance, in intervening years, it has been learned that cognitive impairment is highly prevalent and functionally disruptive and that it occurs in wide-ranging domains. Key questions remain unanswered with regard to vital questions such as determining causes, risk factors, and mechanisms as well as the degree to which brain injuries associated with critical illness are amenable to rehabilitation. Little remains known about the effects of critical illness on elderly ICU cohorts and on the neurologic functioning of individuals with preexisting impairment versus those who are normal. Few data exist regarding the development of strategies designed to prevent the emergence of neuropsychological deficits after critical illness. Although great progress has been made and is ongoing, a pressing need exists for additional investigation of cognitive impairment and other conditions, such as PTSD and quality of life after critical illness, that will seek to untangle the many pertinent questions related to this condition and that will ultimately offer help and hope to the thousands of survivors affected by this condition.

REFERENCES

1. Angus DC, Carlet J. Surviving intensive care: a report from the 2002 Brussels Roundtable. Intensive Care Med 2003;29:368–77.
2. Hopkins RO, Brett S. Chronic neurocognitive effects of critical illness. Curr Opin Crit Care 2005;11(4):369–75.
3. Hopkins RO, Jackson JC. Assessing neurocognitive outcomes after critical illness: are delirium and long-term cognitive impairments related? Curr Opin Crit Care 2006;12:388–94.
4. Hopkins RO, Jackson JC. Long-term neurocognitive function after critical illness. Chest 2006;130(3):869–78.
5. Girard TD, Shintani AK, Jackson JC, et al. Duration of delirium in patients with severe sepsis predicts long-term cognitive impairment. 2006:A739.
6. Pandharipande P, Cotton BA, Shintani A, et al. Prevalence and risk factors for development of delirium in surgical and trauma intensive care unit patients. J Trauma 2008;65(1):34–41.
7. Pandharipande P, Jackson J, Ely EW. Delirium: acute cognitive dysfunction in the critically ill. Curr Opin Crit Care 2005;11(4):360–8.
8. Meagher DJ. Delirium: optimising management. Br Med J 2001;322(7279): 144–9.
9. Lipowski ZJ. Delirium in the elderly patient. N Engl J Med 1989;320(9):578–82.
10. Galanakis P, Bickel H, Gradinger R, et al. Acute confusional state in the elderly following hip surgery: incidence, risk factors and complications. Int J Geriatr Psychiatry 2001;16(4):349–55.
11. O'Keefe ST, Chonchubhair AN. Postoperative delirium in the elderly. Br J Anaesth 1994;73:673–87.
12. Ely EW, Inouye SK, Bernard GR, et al. Delirium in mechanically ventilated patients: validity and reliability of the confusion assessment method for the intensive care unit (CAM-ICU). JAMA 2001;286(21):2703–10.
13. Inouye SK, Rushing JT, Foreman MD, et al. Does delirium contribute to poor hospital outcomes? A three-site epidemiologic study. J Gen Intern Med 1998; 13:234–42.
14. Ely EW, Shintani A, Truman B, et al. Delirium as a predictor of mortality in mechanically ventilated patients in the intensive care unit. JAMA 2004;291(14): 1753–62.
15. ISIS-2. Randomised trial of intravenous streptokinase, oral aspirin, both, or neither among 17187 cases of suspected acute myocardial infarction: ISIS-2. Lancet 1988;2:349–60.
16. Uldall KK, Ryan R, Berghuis JP, et al. Association between delirium and death in AIDS patients. AIDS Patient Care 2000;14:95–100.
17. Eikelenboom P, Hoogendijk WJG. Do delirium and Alzheimer's dementia share specific pathogenetic mechanisms? Dement Geriatr Cogn Disord 1999;10(5): 319–24.
18. Maclullich AM, Beaglehole A, Hall RJ, et al. Delirium and long-term cognitive impairment. Int Rev Psychiatry 2009;21(1):30–42.

19. Jackson JC, Gordon SM, Hart RP, et al. The association between delirium and cognitive decline: a review of the empirical literature. Neuropsychol Rev 2004; 14(2):87–98.

20. Trzepacz PT. Is there a final common neural pathway in delirium? Focus on acetylcholine and dopamine. Semin Clin Neuropsychiatry 2000;5:132–48.

21. Fong TG, Bogardus ST, Daftary A, et al. Cerebral perfusion changes in older delirious patients using 99mTc HMPAO SPECT. J Gerontol A Biol Sci Med Sci 2007; 61A:1294–9.

22. Moody DM, Bell MA, Challa VR. Features of the cerebral vascular pattern that predict vulnerability to perfusion or oxygenation deficiency: an anatomic study. Am J Neuroradiol 2007;11:431.

23. Alexander GE, DeLong MR, Strick PL. Parallel organization of functionally segregated circuits linking basal ganglia and cortex. Annu Rev Neurosci 1986;9: 357–81.

24. Squire L. Declarative and non-declarative memory: multiple brain systems supporting learning and memory. J Cogn Neurosci 1992;4:232–43.

25. Parkin A. Human memory. Curr Biol 1999;9:582–5.

26. Sbordone R, Seyraniniana GD, Ruff RM. Are the subjective complaints of traumatically brain injured patients reliable? Brain Inj 1998;12:505–12.

27. Jackson JC, Gordon SM, Ely EW, et al. Research issues in the evaluation of cognitive impairment in intensive care unit survivors. Intensive Care Med 2004; 30(11):2009–16.

28. Jackson JC, Hart RP, Gordon SM, et al. Six-month neuropsychological outcome of medical intensive care unit patients. Crit Care Med 2003;31(4):1226–34.

29. Hopkins RO, Weaver LK, Pope D, et al. Neuropsychological sequelae and impaired health status in survivors of severe acute respiratory distress syndrome. Am J Respir Crit Care Med 1999;160(1):50–6.

30. Rothenhäusler HB, Ehrentraut S, Stoll C, et al. The relationship between cognitive performance and employment and health status in long-term survivors of the acute respiratory distress syndrome: results of an exploratory study. Gen Hosp Psychiatry 2001;23(2):90–6.

31. Schillerstrom JE, Horton MS, Schillerstorm TL, et al. Prevalence, course, and risk factors for executive impairment in patients hospitalized on a general medical service. Psychosomatics 2007;46:411–7.

32. Schillerstrom JE, Horton MS, Royall DR. The impact of medical illness on executive function. Psychosomatics 2005;46(6):508–16.

33. Hopkins RO, Weaver LK, Collingridge D, et al. Two-year cognitive, emotional, and quality-of-life outcomes in acute respiratory distress syndrome. Am J Respir Crit Care Med 2005;171(4):340–7.

34. Suchyta MR, Hopkins RO, White J, et al. The incidence of cognitive dysfunction after ARDS. Am J Respir Crit Care Med 2004;169:A18.

35. Lyketsos CG, Toone L, Tschanz J, et al. Population-based study of medical comorbidity in early dementia and "cognitive impairment no dementia": association with functional and cognitive impairment - the Cache County Study. Am J Geriatr Psychiatry 2005;13:656–64.

36. Teunissen CE, van Boxtel MP, Bosma H, et al. Inflammation markers in relation to cognition in a healthy aging population. J Neuroimmunol 2003;134(1-2): 142–50.

37. Yaffe K, Lindquist K, Penninx BW, et al. Inflammatory markers and cognition in well-functioning African-American and white elders. Neurology 2003;61(1): 76–80.

38. Hopkins RO, Suchyta MR, Jephson A, et al. Hyperglycemia and neurocognitive outcome in ARDS survivors. Proc Am Thorac Soc 2005;2:A36.
39. Hopkins RO, Weaver LK, Chan KJ, et al. Quality of life, emotional, and cognitive function following acute respiratory distress syndrome. J Int Neuropsychol Soc 2004;10(7):1005–17.
40. Starr JM, Whalley LJ. Drug induced dementia. Drug Saf 1994;11:310–7.
41. Starr JM, Whalley LJ, Deary IJ. The effects of antihypertensive treatment on cognitive function: results from HOPE study. J Am Geriatr Soc 2002;44:411–5.
42. Pomara N, Willoughby L, Wesnes K, et al. Apolipoprotein E epsilon4 allele and lorazepam effects on memory in high-functioning older adults. Arch Gen Psychiatry 2005;62(2):209–16.
43. Kapfhammer HP, Rothenhäusler HB, Krauseneck T, et al. Posttraumatic stress disorder and health-related quality of life in long-term survivors of acute respiratory distress syndrome. Am J Psychiatry 2004;161(1):45–52.
44. Weinert CR, Gross CR, Kangas JR, et al. Health-related quality of life after acute lung injury. Am J Respir Crit Care Med 1997;156:1120–8.
45. Angus D, Musthafa AA, Clermonte G, et al. Quality-adjusted survival in the first year after the acute respiratory distress syndrome. Am J Respir Crit Care Med 2001;163:1389–94.
46. Cheung AM, Tansey CM, Tomlinson G, et al. Two-year outcomes, health care use, and costs of survivors of acute respiratory distress syndrome. Am J Respir Crit Care Med 2006;174(5):538–44.
47. Dowdy DW, Dinglas D, Mendez-Tellez P, et al. Intensive care unit hypoglycemia predicts depression during early recovery from acute lung injury. Crit Care Med 2009;36:2726–33.
48. Katon W, Sullivan MD. Depression and chronic medical illness. J Clin Psychiatry 1990;51:3–11.
49. Silverstone PH. Prevalence of psychiatric disorders in medical illness. J Nerv Ment Dis 1996;184:43–51.
50. Silverstone PH, LeMay T, Elliott J, et al. The prevalence of major depressive disorder and low self esteem in medical inpatients. Can J Psychiatry 1996;41:67–74.
51. Skodol AE. Anxiety in the medically ill: nosology and principles of differential diagnosis. Semin Clin Neuropsychiatry 1999;4:64–71.
52. Nelson BJ, Weinert CR, Bury CL, et al. Intensive care unit drug use and subsequent quality of life in acute lung injury patients. Crit Care Med 2000;28(11):3626–30.
53. Dowdy DW, Bienvenu OJ, Dinglas VD, et al. Are intensive care factors associated with depressive symptoms 6 months after acute lung injury? Crit Care Med 2009;37(5):1702–7.
54. Kress JP, Gehlbach B, Lacy M, et al. The long-term psychological effects of daily sedative interruption on critically ill patients. Am J Respir Crit Care Med 2003;168(12):1457–61.
55. Strain JJ, Liebowithz MR, Klein DF. Anxiety and panic attacks in the medically ill. Psychiatr Clin North Am 1981;4:333–50.
56. Pollack MH, Kradin R, Otto MW. Prevalence of panic in patients referred for pulmonary function testing at a major medical center. Am J Psychiatry 2009;153:110–3.
57. Katz IR. On the inseparability of mental and physical health in aged persons: lesions from depression and medical comorbidity. Am J Geriatr Psychiatry 1996;4:1–16.

58. Jackson JC, Hart RP, Gordon SM, et al. Post-traumatic stress disorder and post-traumatic stress symptoms following critical illness in medical intensive care unit patients: assessing the magnitude of the problem. Crit Care 2007;11(1):R27.
59. Foreman M, Milisen K. Improving recognition of delirium in the elderly. Prim Psychiatry 2004;11:46–50.
60. Sbordone R, Liter J. Mild traumatic brain injury does not produce posttraumatic stress disorder. Brain Inj 1995;9:405–12.
61. Malt L. The long term psychiatric consequences of accidental injury. Br J Psychiatry 1988;153:810–8.
62. Ursano R, Fullerton C, Epstein R. Acute and chronic posttraumatic stress disorder in motor vehicle victims. Am J Psychiatry 1999;156:589–95.
63. Bontke C, Rattok J, Boake C. Do patients with mild brain injury have posttraumatic stress disorder too? J Head Trauma Rehabil 1996;11:95–102.
64. Klein E, Caspi Y, Gil S. The relation between memory of the traumatic brain injury and PTSD: evidence from studies of traumatic brain injury. Can J Psychiatry 2003; 48:28–33.
65. Bryant RA. Posttraumatic stress disorder and traumatic brain injury: can they co-exist? Clin Psychol Rev 2001;21:931–48.
66. Brewin CR. A cognitive neuroscience account of posttraumatic stress disorder and its treatment. Behav Res Ther 2001;39:373–93.
67. Brewin CR, Dalgleish T, Joseph S. A dual representation theory of posttraumatic stress disorder. Psychol Rev 1996;103:670–86.
68. Schacter DL, Chiu CYP, Ochsner KN. Implicit memory: a selective review. Neuroscience 1993;16:159–82.
69. Sessler C. Top ten list in sepsis. Chest 2001;120:1390–3.
70. Jones C, Griffiths RD, Humprhis G. Disturbed memory and amnesia related to intensive care. Memory 2000;8:79–94.
71. Ely EW, Margolin R, Francis J, et al. Evaluation of delirium in critically ill patients: validation of the Confusion Assessment Method for the Intensive Care Unit (CAM-ICU). Crit Care Med 2001;29(7):1370–9.
72. Ely EW, Siegel MD, Inouye SK. Delirium in the intensive care unit: an under-recognized syndrome of organ dysfunction. Semin Respir Crit Care Med 2001; 22(2):115–26.
73. Capuzzo M, Valpondi V, Cingolani E, et al. Post-traumatic stress disorder-related symptoms after intensive care. Minerva Anestesiol 2005;71(4):167–79.
74. Capuzzo M, Valpondi V, Cingolani E, et al. Application of the Italian version of the intensive care unit memory tool in the clinical setting. Crit Care 2004;8(1):R48–55.
75. Jones C, Griffiths RD, Humphris G, et al. Memory, delusions, and the development of acute posttraumatic stress disorder-related symptoms after intensive care. Crit Care Med 2001;29(3):573–80.
76. Jones C, Skirrow P, Griffiths RD, et al. Rehabilitation after critical illness: a randomized, controlled trial. Crit Care Med 2003;31(10):2456–61.
77. Heyland DK, Hopman W, Coo H, et al. Long-term health-related quality of life in survivors of sepsis. Short form 36: a valid and reliable measure of health-related quality of life. Crit Care Med 2000;28:3599–605.
78. Combes A, Costa MA, Trouillet JL, et al. Morbidity, mortality, and quality-of-life outcomes of patients requiring ≥14 days of mechanical ventilation. Crit Care Med 2003;31(5):1373–81.
79. Orme JF, Romney JS, Hopkins RO, et al. Pulmonary function and health-related quality of life in survivors of acute respiratory distress syndrome. Am J Respir Crit Care Med 2003;167:690–4.

80. Herridge MS, Cheung AM, Tansey CM, et al. One-year outcomes in survivors of the acute respiratory distress syndrome. N Engl J Med 2003;348(8):683–93.
81. Dowdy DW, Eid MP, Sedrakyan A, et al. Quality of life in adult survivors of critical illness: a systematic review of the literature. Intensive Care Med 2005;31(5): 611–20.
82. Capes SE, Hunt D, Malmberg K, et al. Stress hyperglycemia and prognosis of stroke in nondiabetic and diabetic patients: a systematic overview. Stroke 2001;32(10):2426–32.
83. Sukantarat KT, Burgess PW, Williamson RC, et al. Prolonged cognitive dysfunction in survivors of critical illness. Anaesthesia 2005;60(9):847–53.
84. Toshima MT, Blumberg E, Ries AL. Does rehabiliation reduce depression in patients with chronic obstructive pulmonary disease? J Cardiopulm Rehabil 1992; 12:261–9.
85. Robertson IH, Murre JM. Rehabilitation of brain damage: brain plasticity and principles of guided recovery. Psychol Bull 1999;125(5):544–75.

Physical and Psychiatric Recovery from Burns

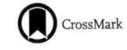

Frederick J. Stoddard Jr, MD[a], Colleen M. Ryan, MD[b], Jeffrey C. Schneider, MD[c],*

KEYWORDS

- Rehabilitation • Resilience • Recovery • Body image • Posttraumatic stress disorder
- Depression • Hypertrophic scar • Burn reconstruction

KEY POINTS

- Burn injuries pose complex biopsychosocial challenges to recovery. A focus of care on rehabilitation and recovery is becoming more important with improved survival rates in the United States.
- The physical and emotional sequelae of burns differ widely, depending on the individual's resilience and the time in the life cycle in which they occur.
- Most burn survivors are resilient and recover, whereas some are more vulnerable and have more complicated biopsychosocial outcomes.
- Physical rehabilitation is affected by pain, orthopedic, neurologic, and metabolic complications.
- Psychiatric recovery is affected by posttraumatic stress disorder, depression, learning disorders, substance abuse, stigma, and disability. Individual resilience, social support, and education or occupation affect outcomes.

INTRODUCTION

Burn injuries pose complex biopsychosocial challenges to recovery. The incidence of burns in the United States has decreased dramatically in the past 50 years as a result of public education and home and work safety devices and regulations. In addition, survival rates have improved significantly.[1] As a result, the need for an emphasis on rehabilitation and recovery is paramount, with special focus on lessening the biopsychosocial impact of burn disfigurement, functional disabilities, mental disorders, and problems at school or work. A key goal is to teach patients and families strategies for successful rehabilitation, how to enhance resilience,[2,3] how to reduce the stigma of

This article first appeared in Surg Clin N Am 2014;94(4):863–878.
^a Department of Psychiatry, Massachusetts General Hospital, Harvard Medical School, Boston, MA, USA; ^b Department of Surgery, Massachusetts General Hospital, Harvard Medical School, Boston, MA, USA; ^c Spaulding Rehabilitation Hospital, Harvard Medical School, 300 1st Avenue, Boston, MA 02129, USA
* Corresponding author.
E-mail address: jcschneider@partners.org

Psychiatr Clin N Am 38 (2015) 105–120
http://dx.doi.org/10.1016/j.psc.2014.11.001
0193-953X/15/$ – see front matter © 2015 Elsevier Inc. All rights reserved.

burns, and help them cope effectively in society.[4] Burn survivors have complicated psychiatric and rehabilitation needs, which are greater for those who are economically disadvantaged or with preexisting psychosocial risks. Their needs include early preventive interventions to reduce the acute physical and psychological trauma of burns and to improve long-term outcomes,[5] such as management of acute pain, stress, and grief, and of longer-term issues such as skin, bone, metabolic, neurologic, pulmonary, and psychiatric disorders, including body image, depression, posttraumatic stress disorder (PTSD), and substance abuse. Although not long ago, little was known about which mental disorders in patients with burns require diagnosis and treatment to improve outcomes, more is known about how they delay or block recovery and how to treat them. Recovery lasts from months to years, often with lifelong sequelae. Optimal long-term care involves a multidisciplinary team, which includes the burn surgeon, plastic/reconstructive surgeon, psychiatrist, physiatrist, psychologist, physical and occupational therapists, nurse, nutritionist, and subspecialists in areas such as pulmonary medicine, orthopedics, infectious disease, ear, nose, and throat, endocrinology, dentistry, and cosmetology.

Developmental Considerations Across the Life Cycle

Burns affect people at any time in life, from earliest infancy to late life.

The physical and emotional sequelae of burns differ widely depending on the individual's resilience, including genetic and genomic risk, and the time of life in which the burns occur. The younger the person, the longer the psychosocial impact of the stigma of burn disfigurement, because there are more remaining life years of potential physical and emotional disability. Nevertheless, the young tend to heal more rapidly overall than the elderly, and have fewer comorbid conditions, so their prognosis for physical and emotional recovery is better for equivalent injuries. Physically, children are growing rapidly, and this may benefit but also complicate healing. Benefits include more rapid healing and usually, greater metabolic resiliency and resistance to infection, whereas complications long-term include scars growing with the child and contractures forming as the child grows in weight and height. Psychologically, children are more likely to have family supports and less apt to have preexisting psychopathology than adults and may therefore adjust more readily; on the other hand, the pain and trauma of burns and burn treatment may affect personality, cognitive, and emotional development for their entire lives, leaving lifelong physical and emotional scars.[6] Infant-parent and child-parent relationships are significantly affected by the stress and stigma of a child's burn on the mother or father, including the inevitable guilt that they carry. Adolescents, who are also growing, are vulnerable to interference in body image development, and in developing self-esteem, mood regulation, cognitive mastery, intellectual development in school, and love relationships. Adults, including the elderly, may heal more slowly and may have to grieve losses of appearance, function, and social/occupational relationships, which have defined them for a lifetime, including the capacity to work. The elderly patient with a severe burn may live alone with few supports and may require extensive rehabilitation and social services to recover as much function as possible with or without continued independent living. As discussed later, some patients do not recover and die. End-of-life care, an essential part of clinical care, is more common in caring for severely burned adults with higher mortality, but is a key clinical skill of staff in both pediatric and adult burn centers.

Psychiatric risks, complications, and treatment

Among the psychosocial risk factors for burns are poverty, abuse and neglect, alcohol and substance abuse, serious mental illness, suicide, and assault. Psychiatric risk requires assessment and alert triage at the time of admission, for possible full psychiatric diagnostic evaluation and treatment. Disorders present at admission for burn injuries or shortly afterward adversely affect long-term outcomes, and suicide may occur. The mental disorders in patients with burns include preexisting mental illness or substance abuse (eg, withdrawal), untreated burn pain syndromes,[7] delirium, sleep disorders, and acute stress disorder and require early diagnosis and treatment to mitigate long-term risks. Occasional patients are burned as a result of a suicide or homicide attempt, and this may not be known initially. During intermediate care, and during burn recovery and rehabilitation, a broader range of psychiatric problems commonly emerge in children or adults, also requiring diagnosis and specific psychiatric or psychological treatment.[8,9] Among this broader range of psychiatric problems are (in young children) separation anxiety, PTSD, and attachment disorders and (in all patients) phantom limb phenomena, affective disorders (major depression or bipolar disorder), attention-deficit/hyperactivity disorder, PTSD, and other anxiety disorders, especially phobias, sleep disorders, autistic spectrum disorders, personality disorders, somatization disorder, and dementia.[8] Learning disabilities are common, in both children and adults with burns, and often interfere, if not recognized, in recovery and in adherence to rehabilitation interventions.

The range of specific therapies is broad, from acute treatments for alcohol or drug withdrawal to psychopharmacology of sleep disorders, psychosis, PTSD, or depression, to individual psychotherapy and family therapy to enhance resilience and reduce the long-term psychological impact of burn trauma and disfigurement.[10] Although most patients recover, some require transfer or referral to long-term outpatient psychiatric treatment, brief inpatient services, or psychological counseling at school or at work.

Disasters present special psychiatric problems; an awareness of these is critical to preparedness of burn centers[10–13] to serve their communities. The surgical and psychiatric responses after the Coconut Grove fire in 1942 in Boston introduced 2 eras: toward both contemporary burn care and toward contemporary disaster psychiatry.[14] Among many essential issues for burn center staffs is advance disaster mental health training, needs assessment, and knowledge of vulnerable populations, and for responders to attend to their own self-care.

Skin Complications: Effects of Thermal Injury, Skin Regeneration, and Scarring

In thermal injury, the extent of tissue damage is related to the location, duration, and intensity (temperature) of heat exposure. After burn injury a cascade of physiologic processes affect the impact of the thermal injuries. Damaged skin results in impairment in most major functions of the integumentary system. In areas of burn injury, skin loses its ability to act as a protective barrier and homeostatic regulator. This situation may lead to significant losses of body fluid, impaired thermoregulation, and increased susceptibility to infection. Spontaneous reepithelialization is impossible with a full-thickness burn injury, because of destruction of the dermal appendages. Full-thickness burns result in hair loss, sensory impairment, loss of normal skin lubrication, and heat intolerance as a result of destruction of sweat glands.

Hypertrophic Scarring

This topic is covered in the article on biology and principles of scar management and burn reconstruction elsewhere in this issue.

Ultraviolet sensitivity and skin pigmentation

Sun protection is essential for burn survivors. The area of burn injury is susceptible to damage from ultraviolet radiation from the sun, regardless of preinjury skin pigmentation.

Burn survivors of deep partial-thickness and full-thickness burns are advised to avoid and protect against sun exposure for the first few years after injury. Avoiding direct sun exposure minimizes risk of sunburn. Covering sites of burn injury with clothing for at least the first year after injury is recommended. In addition, sunscreen with a sun protection factor of 15 or greater should be applied to healed burn sites before any sun exposure.[15] Pigmentation changes are common after burn injury. Studies have shown the development of hyperpigmentation by spectrophotometry measurements at the burn site. Hyperpigmentation correlated with premorbid skin color, age, sun exposure, and time after injury.[16,17] Also, deep partial-thickness and full-thickness burn injuries may result in hypopigmentation or depigmentation. Dyspigmentation after burn injury can be treated surgically. Researchers have reported[18] success in treating hyperpigmented skin grafts of the hand with surgical excision and split-thickness skin grafts and hypopigmented burn sites of the hand with dermabrasion and split-thickness skin grafts. Good results have also been reported[19] treating depigmented burn scar using carbon dioxide laser for dermabrasion followed by split-thickness skin grafting. Malignancy development of malignant tumors in chronic burn scars is rare. Most tumors are squamous cell carcinoma; basal cell carcinoma and malignant melanoma are less common. Diagnosis ranges from 20 to 30 years after burn injury. Two large cohort studies[20,21] followed 16,903 and 37,095 burn survivors, respectively, for a mean of 16 years. There was no increased risk for squamous cell carcinoma, basal cell carcinoma or malignant melanoma in the burn survivors compared with the general population. Subgroup analysis of those with more severe burns and longer follow-up showed no increased risk for skin cancer.

Bone and Joint Changes

Musculoskeletal complications are common after burn injuries. Prevention, early identification, and treatment are the goals of care. Contractures are a major musculoskeletal complication of burn injury and are covered in the article on management of common postburn deformities elsewhere in this issue. Bone and joint changes are addressed in detail in **Table 1**.

Bone metabolism

Delay in bone growth is a complication seen in children after severe burn injury.[22] Growth disturbances result from the premature fusion of the epiphyseal plate of

Table 1 Musculoskeletal complications of burn injuries	
Complication	**Comments**
Changes in bone metabolism	Common in children; premature fusion of epiphyseal plate of long bones; low bone mineral density in large burns
Osteophytes	Most frequent skeletal change; most common at elbow
Heterotopic ossification	Most common at elbow. Risk factors include burn size, ventilator support, intensive care unit stay, prolonged wound closure, wound infection, and graft loss
Scoliosis and kyphosis	Children with asymmetric burns and contractures develop scoliosis and kyphosis
Septic arthritis	Caused by penetrating burns into a joint or hematogenous seeding; associated with joint dislocation, bone and joint destruction, and restriction of movement
Subluxations and dislocations	Most common in hand and feet caused by contracture formation. Prevention with splinting and range of motion

affected long bones. Partial epiphyseal plate fusion may occur as well, causing bone deviation and deformity.[23,24] Bone growth issues should be considered in growing children with burn scars that cross a joint and with joint contractures. In addition, a few case reports have documented pressure garments for treatment of facial burns in children altering facial bone growth. Overbites may develop as a result of excessive pressure on the mandible. It is recommended to closely monitor facial development during and after pressure garment use in children for development of normal dental and facial proportions.[25,26] Pressure garments may need to be modified and changed frequently to avoid these complications.

Children with burns greater than 15% total body surface area (TBSA) have decreased bone mineral density. Investigators[27] found decreased bone mineral density at 8 weeks after injury, and the loss is sustained at 5 years after injury. The mechanism for loss of bone mass likely involves multiple factors, including increase in endogenous glucocorticoids, resorptive cytokines from the systemic inflammatory response, vitamin D deficiency, and disruption of calcium metabolism. Reduced bone density places children at risk for long bone fractures.[28–31] Investigators[32] have studied the use of recombinant human growth hormone, without proven effect on bone formation. Recent studies have reported improved bone mineral density with bisphosphonate therapy. In a randomized controlled trial of children with greater than 40% TBSA,[33,34] acute administration (within 10 days of injury) of intravenous pamidronate resulted in higher whole body and lumbar spine bone mineral content at discharge, 6 months and 2 years compared with controls.

Osteophytes

Osteophytes are the most frequently observed skeletal alteration in adult patients with burns. Osteophytes are most often seen at the elbow and occur along the articular margins of the olecranon or coronoid process[35,36]; they are believed to be caused by superimposed minor trauma to affected areas. Pain and nerve impingement can occur depending on the size and location of the osteophytes.

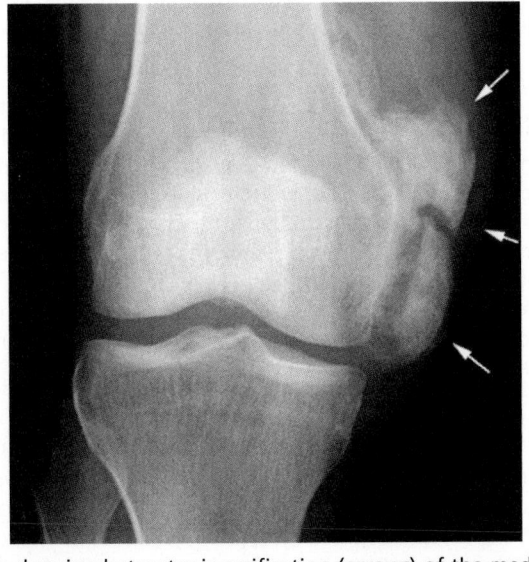

Fig. 1. Radiograph showing heterotopic ossification (*arrows*) of the medial knee.

Heterotopic ossification

Heterotopic ossification (HO) is the abnormal formation of bone in soft tissue (**Fig. 1**). The incidence of HO is estimated at 1% to 2% of hospitalized patients with burns.[37–39] Clinically, only those with symptomatic joints require diagnostic evaluation. Therefore, reports in the literature reflect the incidence of clinically significant HO, not the true incidence. It is postulated[40] that the cause is related to proliferation of mesenchymal cells into osteogenic cells. The elbow is the most frequent joint affected, comprising greater than 90% of cases in a recent review.[39] HO may occur as early as 5 weeks but usually develops approximately 3 months after injury. One of the earliest signs of HO is loss of joint range of motion. Symptoms may precede radiologic findings. A bone scan is the most sensitive diagnostic imaging test and may show positive findings up to 3 weeks before positive radiographic findings[41]; plain radiographs show greater specificity than bone scan.[42]

Treatment of HO begins with conservative measures, including positioning and range of motion to prevent worsening of joint motion. There are no studies examining HO prophylaxis in patients with burns. However, there is evidence to support use of prophylaxis in other conditions, and these data may help guide management of HO in the burn population. Nonsteroidal antiinflammatory drugs (NSAIDs), bisphosphonates, and radiation have proven efficacy for HO prophylaxis in patients with major hip surgery and[43–45] and spinal cord injury.[46,47] Heterotopic bone that causes nerve entrapment requires timely surgery to avoid permanent nerve injury. In the absence of nerve injury, it is common to wait until the bone is mature before surgery. HO matures over approximately 1 year, and serial radiographs are used to monitor for bone stabilization. Surgical excision of HO at the elbow results in improvement in range of motion.[48,49]

Scoliosis and kyphosis

In the growing child, asymmetric burns of the trunk, hips, and shoulder girdle with resultant postural changes and in combination with contracture of burn scars can result in structural scoliosis.[50] Similarly, childhood burns of the anterior neck, shoulders, and chest wall may produce a rounding of the shoulders and sunken chest. Likewise, burn scar shortening and protective posturing can result in kyphosis. It is recommended to have orthopedic surgery follow such patients, because both scoliosis and kyphosis are amenable to bracing and surgical interventions.

Septic arthritis

Septic arthritis is challenging to diagnose in the severely burned patient. The characteristic signs and symptoms are often absent or masked by the overlying burn wound. Joint pain, swelling, color change, and tenderness are common symptoms at the site of burn injury or grafting and therefore are difficult to distinguish from septic arthritis. The 2 major causes of a septic joint are penetrating burns into a joint and hematogenous seeding from bacteremia. Patients with burns are at risk for infection because of their impaired immune system and concurrent illness. Septic arthritis may cause gross dislocation, as a result of capsular laxity or cartilage and bone destruction,[51] or result in severe restriction of movement or ankylosis. It occurs most frequently in the joints of the hands, hips, knees, and wrists.

Subluxation and dislocation

Joint subluxation of the hands and feet is common after burn injury. Burns of the dorsal surface may contract, resulting in joint hyperextension. Prolonged hyperextension places the joint at risk for subluxation. This condition is most common at the metacarpophalangeal (MCP) and metatarsophalangeal (MTP) joints. Ulnar neuropathy places the patient at additional risk for subluxation of the fourth and fifth digits. For dorsal hand burns, prevention of subluxation is achieved with a combination of splinting and range of motion exercises. Splinting places the MCP joints in 60° to 90° of flexion and the distal and proximal interphalangeal joints in full extension. Similarly, the MTP joints may sublux after contracture of healed wounds, especially in children. Application of surgical high-top shoes with a metatarsal bar helps prevent toe deformities. Posterior hip dislocation occurs in children. Hips maintained in an adducted and flexed position are at risk for dislocation. Anterior shoulder dislocations occur in positions of abduction and extension. Shoulder dislocations may result from positioning in the operating room.[52]

Amputation

Deep muscle injury and necrosis occur as a result of deep burn injuries, high-tension electric injuries, and other burn-associated trauma. Bone has a high resistance compared with other tissues, and therefore, a high amount of heat is dissipated in bony areas.[53] Given its proximity to electric current, muscle is predisposed to severe thermal injury, with ensuing necrosis. Muscle necrosis can lead to edema, increase in intracompartment pressure, and subsequent compartment syndrome. The route of electric current often spares the skin that is superficial to muscle necrosis and can lead to unrecognized deep tissue injury. Early escharotomy and fasciotomy may prevent subsequent amputation as a result of compartment syndrome.[54] Significant muscle and tissue necrosis at distal extremities, usually the sites of entry and exit of the electric current, may require amputation.[55,56]

Physical rehabilitation after an amputation is a multistage process, also involving psychological rehabilitation and adaptation to loss of the specific body part, with a goal of maintaining hope for future restoration of function and appearance. Although amputations of the digits or limbs are most common, other body parts may require amputation, such as the nose, ear, breast, or penis. Maturation of a residual limb as well as healing of skin grafts is required before fitting of a definitive prosthesis. Maturation has occurred when postoperative edema has resolved, the volume of the limb has stabilized, and the limb has molded into a cylindrical shape that optimizes prosthetic fitting. Longitudinal prosthetic and physical medicine and rehabilitation care is recommended.

NEUROLOGIC INJURIES

Neurologic complications are often underreported, because the diagnosis is commonly delayed or missed entirely. Assessment is marred by the complexity of medical problems and impaired consciousness of the critically ill patient, but these injuries cause serious debility and functional deficits. Prevention and identification of neuropathies are an important aspect of rehabilitation.

Localized Neuropathies

Localized neuropathies are common, with an incidence of 15% to 37%.[57,58] Electric injury, alcohol abuse, and length of intensive care stay are risk factors for development of mononeuropathies.[59] Premorbid factors such as elderly age and diabetes are risk factors for peripheral nerve compromise.[60] Also, prevention of compression neuropathy is an important tenet of rehabilitation. Bulky dressings can cause compression to superficial peripheral nerves, and improper and prolonged positioning can cause excessive stretch of nerves. Proper positioning and monitoring of wound care can mitigate neurologic complications. Clinical pearls of specific mononeuropathies and brachial plexopathy are reviewed in **Table 2**.

Table 2
Localized neuropathies and associated risk factors

Neuropathy	Risk Factors
Brachial plexus	Shoulder abduction >90°, external rotation Axilla/lateral chest wall grafting position
Ulnar nerve	Elbow flexion 90°, pronation, tourniquet paralysis
Radial nerve	At spiral groove: resting on side rails, hanging over edge of operating table, tourniquet paralysis At wrist: wrist restraints
Median nerve	Edema, prolonged or repeated wrist hyperextension, tourniquet paralysis
Peroneal nerve	Frog leg position, lateral decubitus position, metal stirrups, leg straps, bulky dressings
Femoral nerve	Hematoma at femoral triangle, retroperitoneal bleed

Peripheral Polyneuropathy

Peripheral neuropathy is believed to be caused by a combination of direct thermal injury on the nerves, circulating neurotoxins, and changes in distribution of fluid and electrolytes.[61] Generalized peripheral polyneuropathy is common, with an incidence that ranges from 15% to 30%.[58,60,62] Age and length of intensive care stay are risk factors for developing polyneuropathies.[59] Polyneuropathy is more common in those with greater than 20% TBSA burns and electric injuries.[63–65] Electrophysiologic evidence of polyneuropathy is common within 1 week of severe burn injury.[66] Clinically, patients may have symptoms of paresthesia and signs of mild to moderate weakness in the muscles of the distal extremities. On manual muscle testing, most patients recover their strength, although they may complain of easy fatigability for years after the burn.[57,60,62]

Mononeuritis Multiplex

Mononeuritis multiplex is an asymmetric sensory and motor peripheral neuropathy that involves 2 or more isolated peripheral nerves. It is a common diagnosis in patients with burns with a neuropathy.[65,67]

Pruritus

The mechanism of pruritus is not well understood. Although not as devastating as some other neurologic complications, itch is a significant complaint for many patients. The prevalence of pruritus is as high as 70% at 1 year after injury and has been shown to persist for decades.[68–70] Predictors of pruritus include deep dermal injury, extent of burn, and early posttraumatic stress symptoms.[69,71] A recent review[72] examining pharmacologic and nonpharmacologic treatments of pruritus concluded that interventions lack strong empirical evidence. Nonetheless, there exist multiple clinical treatment options. Nonpharmacologic treatments, including colloidal oatmeal, liquid paraffin, EMLA application (AstraZeneca, Wilmington, DE), pulsed dye laser, silicone gel, scar massage and transcutaneous electric nerve stimulation, have positive effects.[72–74] A mainstay of treatment focuses on use of antihistamines, because histamine, found in abundance in burn wounds, is implicated as a primary mediator of pruritus. Topical medications include histamine receptor antagonists and prudoxin.[75] Oral options also include selective histamine receptor antagonists and prudoxin,[76] as well as recent evidence for use of gabapentin and ondansetron.[77] For those with severe itching, often, a combination of interventions is needed to control symptoms.

PAIN COMPLICATIONS

Pain management after burn injury is an integral part of care and recovery. Background nociceptive pain from the injury itself and exacerbations of pain from intermittent debridement dressing changes or procedures cause significant discomfort. Long-acting opioid pain medications are commonly used to treat the background pain.[78] Premedication with short-acting opioid before dressing changes or procedures and for breakthrough pain is standard care.[79] Because of development of drug tolerance or a history of recreational opioid use, both common in patients with burns, selection of opioids and doses has to be individualized to patients and may exceed standard dosing guidelines. As the wounds heal, a slow and careful opioid taper is needed to prevent withdrawal. Although there is limited evidence for sole use of nonopioids in severe burn pain, NSAIDs and acetaminophen can be valuable, in combination with opioids.[78]

Strong consideration should also be given to nonpharmacologic pain treatment options. Techniques that show reduction of pain scores include massage, hypnosis, multimodal distraction techniques, cognitive-behavioral techniques, and music therapy.[78,80,81] Even off-the-shelf virtual reality can reduce acute pain intensity during wound care procedures.[82] Furthermore, pain is often a multifactorial experience, and therefore, clinicians should make extended efforts to treat all possible contributing causes. These additional factors may include pruritus, neuropathy, anxiety, sleep disturbance, depression, and posttraumatic stress.

Neuropathic pain after burn injury, although not well categorized in the literature, occurs frequently. It is defined as pain initiated or caused by a primary lesion or dysfunction in the peripheral or central nervous system. Neuropathic pain symptoms consisting of pins and needles, burning, stabbing, shooting, or electric sensations are common complaints of patients with burns after healing of their open wounds.[83–85] Treatment includes gabapentin, tricyclic antidepressants, opioids, and steroid injections into hypertrophic scars.

Cognitive Deficits

Cognitive impairments may result from multiple factors associated with burn injury, including anoxia, toxic fume inhalation, and head injury associated with the context of the burn, inhalation injury, hypoperfusion secondary to volume depletion and shock, medical complications from the primary injury such as dehydration and electrolyte abnormalities, and use of centrally acting medications. A high index of suspicion is needed for diagnosis and treatment of patients with mild cognitive impairments. Neuropsychological evaluation may assist in diagnosis, particularly in cases with mild deficits and unclear cause. Speech and language pathology treatment is a useful intervention for cognitive deficits.

METABOLIC COMPLICATIONS
Catabolic State and Exercise

Release of catecholamines plays a key role in the development of a catabolic state after burn injury. Patients with burns greater than 40% TBSA experience a hypermetabolic response for at least 1 year after injury. Catabolism contributes significantly to morbidity and mortality. The catabolic state in burn injury is associated with impaired wound healing, increased infection risk, tachycardia, loss of lean body mass, slowed rehabilitation, and delayed community reintegration. Pharmacologic and nonpharmacologic strategies are implemented to help reverse the effects of catabolism. Nonpharmacologic interventions include early burn wound excision and closure, aggressive treatment of sepsis, maintenance of thermal neutrality by increasing the ambient temperature, high-carbohydrate and high-protein diet, and early institution of resistive exercises. Pharmacologic interventions may include use of recombinant human growth hormone, low-dose insulin infusion, synthetic testosterone analogue (oxandrolone), and β-blockade.[32,86–88] Although individuals with small burns did not differ from those without injury in muscle strength, those with greater than 30% TBSA burns produce less torque, work, and power in their quadriceps when compared with matched controls.[89] A structured exercise program composed of aerobic and resistance training leads to increased function, as measured by increased muscle mass, strength, and cardiovascular endurance. In addition, exercise participants have required significantly fewer surgical releases up to 2 years after the intervention compared with controls.[90] Regular exercise after burn injury, like in other adults, results in improved flexibility, endurance, balance, and strength. Such gains are important for returning to full independence and function. Other benefits of exercise include reduced anxiety and an improved sense of well-being.[91]

The benefits of oxandrolone on hypermetabolism in burn injury have been well supported by multiple well-designed studies in recent years. In a prospective randomized controlled trial of burned children with greater than 40% TBSA burns,[92] patients receiving oxandrolone for at least 7 days during acute hospitalization had shorter length of intensive care unit stay and higher lean body mass than controls. When oxandralone was given to children for 1 year after severe burn, patients had continued improved lean body mass, bone mineral content, muscle strength, height, and weight compared with controls.[93] A separate multicenter prospective randomized controlled trial of adults with 20% to 60% TBSA burns was stopped early because significantly shorter length of stay was shown by the oxandrolone group compared with controls.[94]

Temperature regulation

Full-thickness burns damage the sweat glands of the dermis. Despite treatment with skin grafting, the sweat glands are not replaced or regenerated. Impaired sweating may affect thermoregulation,[95] particularly with those with larger TBSA burns. Patients with large burn injuries often report overheating and increased sweating in areas of unburned skin with exercise and heat.[96] Such complaints may interfere with exercise tolerance, overall fitness, and health, as well as occupational reintegration.[97] Patients with large burns who exercised (mean 49% TBSA), despite a high sweat rate from their unburned skin, were unable to maintain body temperature compared with nonburned control individuals.[98] However, children with large burns seem to tolerate a short duration of moderate exercise without significant changes in core body temperature.[99]

Psychosocial issues

Although some psychosocial issues and impacts were discussed earlier, considerable work in burn rehabilitation has been devoted to these and to many more. One of the most exciting initiatives, informing burn treatment and rehabilitation research and treatment, is creating algorithms assessing quality of life and identifying vulnerability and resiliency outcomes after different burn severities (massive, moderate, and small). Also, there has long been interest in preexisting psychosocial risk factors, and how to best address the varying psychosocial impacts on body image, appearance, and disability of anatomically distinct burns (facial/head, hand, breast, arm/leg, genital, and anal injuries). There is also interest in the specific complexities associated with rehabilitation after tracheostomy and other pulmonary complications. Anthropologists have worked for more than 50 years to understand and seek to lessen the social stigma associated with facial and other visible disfigurement, with recent progress using online cognitive-behavioral interventions to teach patients social skills to apply in specific social situations.[4,100] A neglected but crucial area is how to lessen the adverse impact (including often PTSD) of a burn on the family, including parents, spouse or partner, siblings, and children. Key predictors of outcome include community reintegration, such as return to school or employment. Other psychosocial interventions of possible benefit for many patients and families are alternative therapies (eg, mind/body, or spiritual and religious outreach), if this is not coercive.

The Phoenix Society, the international self-help organization for burn survivors, merits particular mention. It facilitates helpful communication among burn survivors and groups of survivors. It plays a critical ongoing leadership role in educating burn survivors, working with burn centers, organizing the World Burn Conferences, and participating in meetings of the American Burn Association and the International Society for Burn Injuries.

End-of-Life Care and Ethical Considerations

Not all patients survive to progress to recovery and rehabilitation. Compassionate care of the dying patient, and the family anticipating the loss of a loved one, is among the most challenging clinical situations involving all disciplines on the team, and at times, the ethics committee of the hospital. It entails acknowledgment of a decision that the limits of burn treatment have been reached and a shift from the usual focus on burn recovery. In burn centers, patients are often in intensive care, and occasionally do not survive as a result of their injuries. Providing them and their families with optimal, compassionate care at that time is an integral part of clinical care in all burn centers and involves the patient, the family, the physician, the burn team, and pastoral care. Arriving at decisions and a shared, understood plan of when and how to continue care and when not to, when and how to plan not to resuscitate or to discontinue life-saving measures is a key aspect of care, although less common in the United States, because of improved burn survival. Although this change of direction can be stressful for families, and for burn teams trained to save lives, skill in communication and planning in end-of-life care is also essential to optimal care.

SUMMARY

Burn injuries pose complex biopsychosocial challenges to recovery, which is increasingly a focus of improved comprehensive care. Both burn prevention and burn survival in the United States have improved. The physical and emotional sequelae of burns differ widely, depending on burn severity, individual resilience, and stage of development when they occur. Most burn survivors are resilient and recover, whereas some are more vulnerable and have complicated outcomes. Physical rehabilitation is affected by orthopedic, neurologic, and metabolic complications and disabilities. Psychiatric recovery is affected by pain, mental disorders, substance abuse, and burn stigmatization. Individual resilience, social supports, and educational or occupational achievements affect outcomes. When it is determined that the limits of acute burn care are reached, compassionate end-of-life care is integral to optimal care of the individual and family.

REFERENCES

1. Ryan CM, Schoenfeld DA, Thorpe WP, et al. Objective estimates of the probability of death from burn injuries. N Engl J Med 1998;338:362–6.
2. Charney DS. Psychobiological mechanisms of resilience and vulnerability: implications for successful adaptation to extreme stress [review]. Am J Psychiatry 2004;161:195–216.

3. Friedman MJ. The role of pharmacotherapy in early interventions. In: Blumenfeld M, Ursano RJ, editors. Intervention and resilience after mass trauma. Cambridge (England): Cambridge University Press; 2008. p. 107–25.
4. Bessel A, Brough V, Clarke A, et al. Evaluation of the effectiveness of Face IT, a computer-based psychosocial intervention for disfigurement-related distress. Psychology. Psychol Health Med 2012;17(5):556–77.
5. Pruitt BA Jr, Goodwin CW, Mason AD Jr. Epidemiological, demographic and outcome characteristics of burn injury. In: Herndon DN, editor. Total burn care. 2nd edition. New York: WB Saunders; 2002. p. 16–30.
6. Stoddard FJ. Care of infants, children and adolescents with burn injuries. In: Lewis M, editor. Child and adolescent psychiatry. 3rd edition. Baltimore (MD): Lippincott Williams & Wilkins; 2002. p. 1188–208.
7. Stoddard FJ, Sheridan RL, Martyn JA, et al. Pain management. In: Ritchie EC, editor. Combat and operational behavioral health. In: Lenhart MK, editor. The textbooks of military medicine. . Washington, DC: Department of the Army, Office of The Surgeon General, Borden Institute; 2011. p. 339–58.
8. Stoddard FJ, Levine JB, Lund K. Burn injuries. In: Blumenfield M, Strain J, editors. Psychosomatic medicine. Baltimore (MD): Lippincott Williams & Wilkins; 2006. p. 309–36.
9. American Psychiatric Association. Diagnostic and statistical manual of mental disorders. 5th edition. Washington, DC: American Psychiatric Association; 2013.
10. Stoddard FJ. Outcomes of traumatic exposure. In: Cozza S, Cohen J, Dougherty J, editors. Disaster and trauma, child and adolescent psychiatry clinics of North America. Philadelphia: WB Saunders; 2014. p. 243–56.
11. Stoddard FJ, Pandya A, Katz CL, editors. Disaster psychiatry: readiness, evaluation and treatment. Washington, DC: American Psychiatric Press; 2011.
12. North CS, Pfefferbaum B. Mental health response to community disasters: a systematic review. JAMA 2013;310(5):507–18.
13. Stoddard FJ, Simon NM, Pitman RK. Trauma- and stressor-related disorders. In: Hales RE, Yudofsky S, Roberts L, editors. American psychiatric publishing textbook of psychiatry. 6th edition. American Psychiatric Press; 2014. p. 455–98.
14. Cobb S, Lindemann E. Neuropsychiatric observations after the Coconut Grove fire. Ann Surg 1943;117:814–24.
15. Poh-Fitzpatrick MB. Skin care of the healed burned patient. Clin Plast Surg 1992;19:745–51.
16. deChalain TM, Tang C, Thomson HG. Burn area color changes after superficial burns in childhood: can they be predicted? J Burn Care Rehabil 1998;19:39–49.
17. Carvalho DA, Mariani U, Gomez DS, et al. A study of the post-burned restored skin. Burns 1999;25:385–94.
18. Al-Qattan MM. Surgical management of post-burn skin dyspigmentation of the upper limb. Burns 2000;26:581–6.
19. Acikel C, Ulkur E, Guler MM. Treatment of burn scar depigmentation by carbon dioxide laser-assisted dermabrasion and thin skin grafting. Plast Reconstr Surg 2000;105:1973–8.
20. Mellemkjaer L, Holmich LR, Gridley G, et al. Risks for skin and other cancers up to 25 years after burn injuries. Epidemiology 2006;17:668–73.
21. Lindelof B, Krynitz B, Granath F, et al. Burn injuries and skin cancer: a population-based cohort study. Acta Derm Venereol 2008;88:20–2.
22. Prelack K, Dwyer J, Dallal GE, et al. Growth deceleration and restoration after serious burn injury. J Burn Care Res 2007;28(2):262–8.
23. MacG JD. Destructive burns: some orthopaedic complications. Burns 1980; 7(2):105–22.

24. Reed MH. Growth disturbances in the hands following thermal injuries in children. 2. Frostbite. Can Assoc Radiol J 1988;39(2):95–9.
25. Leung KS, Cheng JC, Ma GF, et al. Complications of pressure therapy for post-burn hypertrophic scars. Biomechanical analysis based on 5 patients. Burns Incl Therm Inj 1984;10(6):434–8.
26. Fricke NB, Omnell ML, Dutcher KA, et al. Skeletal and dental disturbances in children after facial burns and pressure garment use: a 4-year follow-up. J Burn Care Rehabil 1999;20(3):239–49.
27. Klein GL, Herndon DN, Langman CB, et al. Long-term reduction in bone mass after severe burn injury in children. J Pediatr 1995;126(2):252–6.
28. Klein GL, Herndon DN, Goodman WG, et al. Histomorphometric and biochemical characterization of bone following acute severe burns in children. Bone 1995;17(5):455–60.
29. Klein GL, Langman CB, Herndon DN. Vitamin D depletion following burn injury in children: a possible factor in post-burn osteopenia. J Trauma 2002;52(2): 346–50.
30. Klein GL, Bi LX, Sherrard DJ, et al. Evidence supporting a role of glucocorticoids in short-term bone loss in burned children. Osteoporos Int 2004;15(6): 468–74.
31. Mayes T, Gottschlich M, Scanlon J, et al. Four-year review of burns as an etiologic factor in the development of long bone fractures in pediatric patients. J Burn Care Rehabil 2003;24(5):279–84.
32. Klein GL, Wolf SE, Langman CB, et al. Effects of therapy with recombinant human growth hormone on insulin-like growth factor system components and serum levels of biochemical markers of bone formation in children after severe burn injury. J Clin Endocrinol Metab 1998;83:21–4.
33. Klein GL, Wimalawansa SJ, Kulkarni G, et al. The efficacy of acute administration of pamidronate on the conservation of bone mass following severe burn injury in children: a double-blind, randomized, controlled study. Osteoporos Int 2005;16(6):631–5.
34. Przkora R, Herndon DN, Sherrard DJ, et al. Pamidronate preserves bone mass for at least 2 years following acute administration for pediatric burn injury. Bone 2007;41(2):297–302.
35. Evans EB, Smith JR. Bone and joint changes following burns; a roentgenographic study; preliminary report. J Bone Joint Surg Am 1959;41(5):785–99.
36. Evans E. Bone and joint changes secondary to burns. In: Lewis SR, editor. Symposium on the treatment of burns. St Louis (MO): CV Mosby; 1973. p. 76–8.
37. Elledge ES, Smith AA, McManus WF, et al. Heterotopic bone formation in burned patients. J Trauma 1988;28(5):684–7.
38. Peterson SL, Mani MM, Crawford CM, et al. Postburn heterotopic ossification: insights for management decision making. J Trauma 1989;29(3):365–9.
39. Hunt JL, Arnoldo BD, Kowalske K, et al. Heterotopic ossification revisited: a 21-year surgical experience. J Burn Care Res 2006;27(4):535–40.
40. Urist MR, Nakagawa M, Nakata N, et al. Experimental myositis ossificans: cartilage and bone formation in muscle in response to a diffusible bone matrix-derived morphogen. Arch Pathol Lab Med 1978;102(6):312–6.
41. van Kuijk AA, Geurts AC, van Kuppevelt H. Neurogenic heterotopic ossification in spinal cord injury. Spinal Cord 2002;40(7):313–26.
42. Freed JH, Hahn H, Menter R, et al. The use of the three-phase bone scan in the early diagnosis of heterotopic ossification and in the evaluation of didronel therapy. Paraplegia 1982;4:208–16.

43. Schmidt SA, Kjaesgaard-Anderson P, Pederson NW, et al. The use of indomethacin to prevent the formation of heterotopic bone after total hip replacement. A randomized, double-blind clinical trial. J Bone Joint Surg Am 1988;70(6):834–8.

44. Pellegrini VD Jr, Gregoritch SJ. Preoperative irradiation for prevention of heterotopic ossification following total hip arthroplasty. J Bone Joint Surg Am 1996; 78(6):870–81.

45. Neal BC, Rodgers A, Clark T, et al. A systematic survey of 13 randomized trials of non-steroidal anti-inflammatory drugs for the prevention of heterotopic bone formation after major hip surgery. Acta Orthop Scand 2000;71(2):122–8.

46. Finerman GA, Stover SL. Heterotopic ossification following hip replacement or spinal cord injury. Two clinical studies with EHDP. Metab Bone Dis Relat Res 1981;3(4–5):337–42.

47. Banovac K, Williams JM, Patrick LD, et al. Prevention of heterotopic ossification after spinal cord injury with COX-2 selective inhibitor (rofecoxib). Spinal Cord 2004;42(12):707–10.

48. Gaur A, Sinclair M, Caruso E, et al. Heterotopic ossification around the elbow following burns in children: results after excision. J Bone Joint Surg Am 2003; 85(8):1538–43.

49. Tsionos I, Leclercq C, Rochet JM. Heterotopic ossification of the elbow in patients with burns. Results after early excision. J Bone Joint Surg Br 2004; 86(3):396–403.

50. Qiu Y, Wang SF, Wang B, et al. Adolescent scar contracture scoliosis caused by back scalding during the infantile period. Eur Spine J 2007;16(10):1557–62.

51. Kim A, Palmieri TL, Greenhalgh DG, et al. Septic hip presenting with dislocation as a source of occult infection in a burn patient. J Burn Care Res 2006;27(5): 749–52.

52. Hinton AE, King D. Anterior shoulder dislocation as a complication of surgery for burns. Burns 1989;15(4):248–9.

53. Chilbert M, Maiman D, Sances A Jr, et al. Measure of tissue resistivity in experimental electrical burns. J Trauma 1985;25(3):209–15.

54. Kopp J, Loos B, Spilker G, et al. Correlation between serum creatinine kinase levels and extent of muscle damage in electrical burns. Burns 2004;30(7): 680–3.

55. Vrabec R, Kolar J. Bone changes caused by electrical current. In: Transactions of the Fourth International Congress of plastic and reconstructive surgery. Rome (Italy): Excerpta Medica; 1969. p. 215–7.

56. Rai J, Jeschke MG, Barrow RE, et al. Electrical injuries: a 30-year review. J Trauma 1999;46(5):933–6.

57. Henderson B, Koepke GH, Feller I. Peripheral polyneuropathy among patients with burns. Arch Phys Med Rehabil 1971;52(4):149–51.

58. Helm PA, Johnson ER, Carlton AM. Peripheral neurological problems in the acute burn patient. Burns 1977;3(2):123–5.

59. Kowalske K, Holavanahalli R, Helm P. Neuropathy after burn injury. J Burn Care Rehabil 2001;22:353–7.

60. Lee MY, Liu G, Kowlowitz V, et al. Causative factors affecting peripheral neuropathy in burn patients. Burns 2009;35(3):412–6.

61. Jackson L, Keats AS. Mechanism of brachial plexus palsy following anesthesia. Anesthesiology 1965;26:190–4.

62. Helm P. Neuromuscular considerations. In: Helm PA, Fisher SV, editors. Comprehensive rehabilitation of burns. Baltimore (MD): Williams and Wilkins; 1984. p. 235–41.

63. Grube BJ, Heimbach DM, Engrav LH, et al. Neurologic consequences of electrical burns. J Trauma 1990;30(3):254–8.
64. Marquez S, Turley JJ, Peters WJ. Neuropathy in burn patients. Brain 1993; 116(2):471–83.
65. Khedr EM, Khedr T, el-Oteify MA, et al. Peripheral neuropathy in burn patients. Burns 1997;23(7–8):579–83.
66. Margherita AJ, Robinson LR, Heimbach DM. Burn-associated peripheral polyneuropathy. A search for causative factors. Am J Phys Med Rehabil 1995; 74(1):28–32.
67. Dagum AB, Peters WJ, Neligan PC, et al. Severe multiple mononeuropathy in patients with major thermal burns. J Burn Care Rehabil 1993;14(4):440–5.
68. Willebrand M, Low A, Dyster-Aas J, et al. Pruritus, personality traits and coping in long-term follow-up of burn-injured patients. Acta Derm Venereol 2004;84(5): 375–80.
69. Van Loey NE, Bremer M, Faber AW, et al. Itching following burns: epidemiology and predictors. Br J Dermatol 2008;158(1):95–100.
70. Holavanahali RK, Helm PA, Kowalske KJ. Long term outcomes in patients surviving large burns: the skin. J Burn Care Res 2010;31:631–9.
71. Vitale MC, Fields-Blache C, Luterman A. Severe itching in the patient with burns. J Burn Care Rehabil 1991;12(4):330–3.
72. Bell PL, Gabriel V. Evidence based review for the treatment of post-burn pruritus. J Burn Care Res 2009;30(1):55–61.
73. Matheson JD, Clayton J, Muller MJ. The reduction of itch during burn wound healing. J Burn Care Rehabil 2001;22(1):76–81.
74. Hettrick HH, O'Brien K, Laznick H, et al. Effect of transcutaneous electrical nerve stimulation for the management of burn pruritus: a pilot study. J Burn Care Rehabil 2004;25(3):236–40.
75. Eschler DC, Klein PA. An evidence-based review of the efficacy of topical antihistamines in the relief of pruritus. J Drugs Dermatol 2010;9(8):992–7.
76. Pour-Reza-Gholi F, Nasrollahi A, Firouzan A, et al. Low-dose doxepin for treatment of pruritus in patients on hemodialysis. Iran J Kidney Dis 2007;1(1): 34–7.
77. Goutos I, Dziewulski P, Richardson PM. Pruritus in burns: review article. J Burn Care Res 2009;30(2):221–8.
78. Patterson DR, Hofland HW, Espey K, et al. Pain management. Burns 2004;30(8): A10–5.
79. Finn J, Wright J, Fong J, et al. A randomised crossover trial of patient controlled intranasal fentanyl and oral morphine for procedural wound care in adult patients with burns. Burns 2004;30:262–8.
80. Frenay MC, Faymonville ME, Devlieger S, et al. Psychological approaches during dressing changes of burned patients: a prospective randomised study comparing hypnosis against stress reducing strategy. Burns 2001;27:793–9.
81. Sen S, Greenhalgh D, Palmieri T. Review of burn research for the year 2010. J Burn Care Res 2012;33(5):577–86.
82. Kipping B, Rodger S, Miller K, et al. Virtual reality for acute pain reduction in adolescents undergoing burn wound care: a prospective randomized controlled trial. Burns 2012;38(5):650–7.
83. Choiniere M, Melzack R, Papillon J. Pain and paresthesia in patients with healed burns: an exploratory study. J Pain Symptom Manage 1991;6:437–44.
84. Malenfant A, Forget R, Papillon J, et al. Prevalence and characteristics of chronic sensory problems in burn patients. Pain 1996;67:493–500.

85. Schneider JC, Harris NL, El Shami A, et al. A descriptive review of neuropathic-like pain after burn injury. J Burn Care Res 2006;27:524–8.
86. Herndon DN, Hart DW, Wolf SE, et al. Reversal of catabolism by beta-blockade after severe burns. N Engl J Med 2001;345:1223–9.
87. Herndon DN, Tompkins RG. Support of the metabolic response to burn injury. Lancet 2004;363:1895–902.
88. Pereira CT, Herndon DN. The pharmacologic modulation of the hypermetabolic response to burns. Adv Surg 2005;39:245–61.
89. St-Pierre DM, Choiniere M, Forget R, et al. Muscle strength in individuals with healed burns. Arch Phys Med Rehabil 1998;79:155–61.
90. Celis MM, Suman OE, Huang TT, et al. Effect of a supervised exercise and physiotherapy program on surgical interventions in children with thermal injury. J Burn Care Rehabil 2003;24:57–61.
91. Pate RR, Pratt M, Blair SN, et al. Physical activity and public health. A recommendation from the Centers for Disease Control and Prevention and the American College of Sports Medicine. JAMA 1995;273:402–7.
92. Jeschke MG, Finnerty CC, Suman OE, et al. The effect of oxandrolone on the endocrinologic, inflammatory, and hypermetabolic responses during the acute phase postburn. Ann Surg 2007;246:351–60 [discussion: 360–2].
93. Przkora R, Herndon DN, Suman OE, et al. Beneficial effects of extended growth hormone treatment after hospital discharge in pediatric burn patients. Ann Surg 2006;243:796–801 [discussion: 801–3].
94. Wolf SE, Edelman LS, Kemalyan N, et al. Effects of oxandrolone on outcome measures in the severely burned: a multicenter prospective randomized double-blind trial. J Burn Care Res 2006;27:131–9 [discussion: 140–1].
95. Davis SL, Shibasaki M, Low DA, et al. Impaired cutaneous vasodilation and sweating in grafted skin during whole-body heating. J Burn Care Res 2007;28:427–34.
96. Austin KG, Hansbrough JF, Dore C, et al. Thermoregulation in burn patients during exercise. J Burn Care Rehabil 2003;24:9–14.
97. Esselman PC, Askay SW, Carrougher GJ, et al. Barriers to return to work after burn injuries. Arch Phys Med Rehabil 2007;88:S50–6.
98. Shapiro Y, Epstein Y, Ben-Simchon C, et al. Thermoregulatory responses of patients with extensive healed burns. J Appl Physiol Respir Environ Exerc Physiol 1982;53:1019–22.
99. McEntire SJ, Herndon DN, Sanford AP, et al. Thermoregulation during exercise in severely burned children. Pediatr Rehabil 2006;9:57–64.
100. Lansdown R, Rumsey N, Bradbury E, et al. Visibly different: coping with disfigurement. Oxford (England): Butterworth Heinemann; 1997. p. 254.

The Future of the Psychiatric Mental Health Clinical Nurse Specialist
Evolution or Extinction

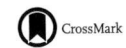

Anita Dempsey, PhD, APRN, PMHCNS-BC*,
Judy Ribak, PhD, APRN, PMHCNS-BC

KEYWORDS

- Psychiatric clinical nurse specialist • Certification • Future role
- Advanced practice registered nurse

KEY POINTS

- The psychiatric mental health clinical nurse specialist (PMHCNS) was the first clinical nurse group to establish specialty certification.
- The role of the PMHCNS includes education in social and psychological models, theory, and individual and group psychotherapeutic treatment methods necessary for comprehensive treatment.
- Although the PMHCNS certification examination will be retired in 2014, other groups can be brought into a similar role through mentoring or expanding the scope of practice.

The role of the psychiatric mental health clinical nurse specialist (PMHCNS) is now in a precarious position. At first glance, some may say it is on the verge of extinction. Because fewer individuals select the specialty option of PMHCNS and in an attempt of the American Nurses Credentialing Center (ANCC) to support the Consensus Model for advanced practice registered nurse (APRN) regulation recommendations (2008),[1] the ANCC has announced that as of 2014 the certification examination for the PMHCNS will be retired.[2] Those currently holding PMHCNS certification have been assured of the ability to continue to practice in the PMHCNS advanced role, as long as all certification renewal requirements regarding professional development activities and clinical practice hours are met in accordance with individual state licensure requirements. However, any lapse in certification may result in the loss of ability to renew

This article first appeared in Nurs Clin N Am 2012;47:295–304.
College of Nursing and Health, Wright State University, 3640 Colonel Glenn Highway, Dayton, OH 45435-0001, USA
* 7660 Burlinehills Court, Cincinnati, OH 45244.
E-mail address: anita.dempsey@wright.edu

Psychiatr Clin N Am 38 (2015) 121–130
http://dx.doi.org/10.1016/j.psc.2014.11.008
0193-953X/15/$ – see front matter © 2015 Elsevier Inc. All rights reserved.

certification and, subsequently, the license to practice as an APRN.[2] This is an alarming message to the PMHCNS, and it certainly indicates a change for this advanced practice nursing role. This change will most certainly lead to the eventual extinction of the originally conceived and currently practiced PMHCNS. As we prepare to implement this sweeping change, it is crucial that the role of the PMHCNS be fully understood so that critical functions do not fall by the wayside. In this article, a brief history of the role of the PMHCNS is reviewed along with current education, practice, role, and ANCC certification of the PMHCNS. The future implications and considerations of the unique functions of the PMHCNS for an APRN with a psychiatric mental health specialization are discussed.

HISTORY

Historically, psychiatric/mental health nurses have been nursing leaders and entrepreneurs. Psychiatric/mental health nurses, in the 1950s, recognized the need for educational and clinical criteria to function as a clinical nurse specialist (CNS), and were the first clinical nursing group to establish certification at the specialist level.[3] The scope of education and practice for the PMHCNS included social and psychological models; a variety of theoretical frameworks to facilitate the understanding of individuals, groups, and systems; and a variety of individual and group psychotherapeutic treatment modalities to support comprehensive treatment and consultation. During the 1980s, an influx of newly prepared CNSs, eager to practice in specialty areas, provided expert clinical care in acute and private settings, consultation services, staff and consumer education, and clinical leadership, and participated in the generation of evidence as a means to achieve the goal of improved outcomes of patient care. Advanced practice nurses, engaged in the role of the PMHCNS, contributed considerably to the quality and continuity of care for patients and family systems in both inpatient and outpatient practice settings. The aim of the PMHCNS has always been to assist the patient to achieve the highest possible level of wellness.

As the role of the PMHCNS emerged, each practitioner modeled the role within the parameters of traditional areas of practice with attention to the needs of the organization and environment of patient care. The PMHCNS became a valued resource providing education, clinical supervision, and mentoring for staff nurses as well as for other professionals within the environment of patient care. Over a period, PMHCNS roles were implemented and interpreted by those who fulfilled the roles to include focus on the treatment of individuals with complex mental health problems, often superimposed upon by both physical health problems and overwhelming psychosocial concerns. The PMHCNS provided the patient (and family) the increased time, attention, and support that physicians did not provide because the physician's traditional focus had been the patient's chief complaint or acute health problem at hand. The PMHCNS was the professional group that forged therapeutic relationships and helped form alliances with individuals and families who needed holistic care to both treat the acute health problem and intervene to address the accompanying psychosocial concern. The PMHCNS had very efficiently developed an independent and complementary role in the treatment of individuals with complex mental health problems, not as a physician extender, but as a holistic care provider with a nursing perspective.

Peplau[4] was clairvoyant in her assumption that the CNS could achieve expertise in the care of individuals with complex health concerns, and in treating the individual and family from a nursing perspective as opposed to the care offered by traditional medicine. Practicing alongside other mental health professionals, in all health care venues, the PMHCNS became the go-to practitioner for expert clinical care, consultation, education, clinical leadership, and research activities. The broad knowledge base, which integrated the physical with the psychosocial, provided a unique and valuable perspective to members of mental health treatment teams as well as to health care system administrators struggling to maintain quality in the rapidly changing health care environment.

CURRENT CNS PRACTICE AND PREPARATION

According to the 2009 Role Delineation Study, there are currently an estimated 6624 PMHCNSs.[5] At the time of the survey, 65% of the participants were 55 years or older, 90% had 20 or more years of experience as a registered nurse, and 80% had been certified as a PMHCNS for 10 or more years.[6] Thus, current PMHCNSs appear to be an older group with a lot of experience. However, as noted in the 2009 Role Delineation Study,[5,6] there has been a decline in individuals taking the PMHCNS certification examination. In 2010, a total of 82 individuals passed the ANCC adult psychiatric mental health certification examination. By contrast, 302 individuals passed the family psychiatric and mental health nurse practitioner (FPMHNP) certification, and 384 individuals passed the adult psychiatric mental health nurse practitioner certification.[6]

The current PMHCNS is the clinical expert at the advanced practice level of care. Inseparable and embedded in the current role are all the functions as originally indicated by the PMHCNS preparation. The PMHCNS is a practitioner who not only defines the diagnosis but also uses multiple modalities to provide patient care, practicing in specialty areas to provide expert clinical care including medication, psychotherapy, consultation services, staff and consumer education, clinical leadership, and generation of evidence. Consider the role of the PMHCNS in the following case.

The patient was an 86-year-old woman, living alone, who had fallen in her home. She had 3 grown-up children, living out of town, who were busy with careers and families of their own. One of the daughters was unable to reach her mother on the phone for 24 hours, and became worried, so she phoned the neighbor who went over to look in on the patient. The patient had been down for at least 10 hours. After an evaluation by the emergency department, the patient had been hospitalized in a senior adult mental health unit, with change in mental status, weight loss, gait disturbance, and possible dysphagia. Two of the daughters came to their mother's side within hours. They were both quite concerned that there had been a dramatic decline in their mother's condition since their most recent visit 4 months ago. Although the patient was glad to see both daughters, there had certainly been a memory decline, difficulty in finding words, and dramatic weight loss.

The PMHCNS met with the patient to complete a baseline evaluation of mental status as well as to obtain the history, current health problems, medication profile, and patient's perception of the current problem. The PMHCNS then met with the daughters to ascertain some of the same information, realizing that the daughters did not have daily or immediate contact with their mother. The PMHCNS investigated current health problems, medications, and treatments with the primary care physician. The gait disturbance was neither reported nor treated previously, and there was also no previously documented concern of confusion in this patient.

The PMHCNS made daily rounds to reassess the patient as well as to keep current on her hospital course, including multidisciplinary assessments and treatments, laboratory results, and diagnostic testing. The patient was found to have global cognitive loss as well as associated gait disturbance and dysphagia. After consultation with the unit nursing staff, occupational therapist, primary care physician, psychiatrist, gastroenterologist, physical therapist, and speech therapist, the PMHCNS prepared a comprehensive report including potential paths for the continued care of the patient.

The primary care physician recommended assisted living; the physical therapist recommended use of a walker and a structured exercise program; the psychiatrist recommended adding an antidepressant; the speech therapist recommended thickening liquids to increase safety in swallowing; the occupational therapist recommended structured recreational activity; and the gastroenterologist recommended permanent insertion of a gastrointestinal tube to provide nutrition, which would eliminate the possibility of aspiration when feeding by mouth.

The PMHCNS called a family meeting and invited the professionals as well as the patient and her children. The patient and her daughters were anxious to hear recommendations for restoring the good health that the patient had enjoyed nearly all her life. The family meeting was conducted by the PMHCNS, who began by exploring with the daughters the changes they found in their mother just before this admission. Each specialist (who attended) presented assessment findings and recommendations for the patient; the CNS then aptly explained the findings of those who were not present, in addition to the psychiatric findings, and invited questions.

The daughters were pleased by the recommendations of each specialist and were eager to proceed with every recommendation on their mother's behalf. The patient, however, was not very pleased about all the changes, including the recommendation to shift her residence and insert a feeding tube. "But mother, as soon as you accept these recommendations, you will feel better again, you will be walking more safely, and you will be back to your old self!" her daughter exclaimed.

The PMHCNS, alerted by the false promise that "you will be back to your old self," asks the daughter to elaborate. The CNS is an expert in providing care and is also alert to unspoken messages communicated in meeting with families, readily able to correct misperceptions and provide in-depth explanation. The feeding tube, for example, would not prevent all aspiration, though it would prevent aspiration from oral intake. The gait disorder would not be resolved by implementation of the exercises and walker; however, the patient would be safer only if she used the assistive device appropriately. There are implications when shifting the residence of a frail individual; the CNS addressed these implications as well. Group psychotherapy skills were used during this meeting; consultation with the family occurred on an ongoing basis during every step of the hospitalization; the multidisciplinary staff was apprised of the patient's and family's course during the hospitalization; clinical leadership was demonstrated as the CNS modeled communication with the patient, family, and multidisciplinary team. The CNS debriefed the nursing staff regarding this patient's care because the patient's primary care nurse was upset at the notion of placing a feeding tube. "Why can't they simply allow her to eat, if she enjoys food?" the distressed staff nurse asked. The CNS provided support for the nurse's concerns, because she used evidence to demonstrate the signs of dysphagia on using the feeding tube. "You are so correct, evidence supports that a patient may continue to aspirate despite insertion of a feeding tube, and the patient and her family now understand this," the CNS replied.

This simulated case demonstrates the expanded practice role that the PMHCNS implements every day. Debriefing the staff regarding the care of the patient, care of families facing the changing health of a member, and interpretation of the tests and procedures are all within the purview of the CNS. The comprehensive nature of care represented by this patient's experiences represents the relationships and roles of the PMHCNS. The role is crucial to both exemplary patient/family care as well as model communication among the disciplines.

Despite the ability to manage complex patient/family situations and to work with a variety of professionals, the ANCC certification criteria for a PMHCNS are the least rigorous when viewed alongside the ANCC certification criteria for the psychiatric and Mental Hhealth Nnurse Ppractitioner (PMHNP) and FPMHNP. Although the PMHCNS criteria were the first developed, they do not seem to fully reflect the many facets of the PMHCNS role. The requirement for the PMHCNS to have education regarding health promotion, disease prevention, differential diagnosis, and disease management is not specified. These functions, however, have for several years been a part of the PMHCNS role and educational curricula. All roles require a minimum of 500 supervised clinical hours and clinical training in 2 psychotherapeutic specialties. It is clear in hindsight that the current PMHCNS certification did not reflect, and currently does not reflect, the scope, skills, knowledge, and value of the historical role of the PMHCNS. Although at first glance there appear to be equal clinical requirements for these 3 certifications, it is worth pointing out that the broader the scope of practice, the more content the 500 supervised clinical hours needs to cover. Thus, the PMHCNS has a more focused clinical experience on aspects of psychiatric mental health in the CNS role, including direct patient care with individuals and families, staff development, clinical supervision, research activities, group facilitation, and consultation, in addition to organizational and systems issues. The PMHNP is focused on providing physical and mental health care to the individual whereas the FPMHNP is focused on providing physical and mental health care to the individual and family, irrespective of age. The broader the clinical scope, the narrower the clinical focus that is concentrated on psychiatric mental health.

The education to become a PMHCNS shows a great degree of variability and flux. While these programs prepare one for practice, they must also prepare one to meet the ANCC certification requirements. A review of a limited sample of study programs that prepare advanced practice nurses for the PMHCNS or PMHNP role (**Table 1**) shows great variability in how these roles are conceptualized. Several individuals identify the role of the PMHCNS as different from that of the PMHNP, by virtue of the focus of the PMHNP on provision of direct patient care, including prescription of medication and interpretation of diagnostic testing. Psychotherapy, a part of the PMHCNS role, is not necessarily seen to be within the scope of the PMHNP practice by some, but is seen to be so by others. Other than for direct patient care, there is little description to support multiple practice roles in the current role of the PMHNP. Collaborative, mentoring, group-facilitating, and interdisciplinary roles are not clearly defined by the PMHNP by program descriptions. Contrary to what the CNS role defines, the PMHNP role does not emphasize care of the family or case management. Clinical supervision of clinical providers is not an indicated skill of the PMHNP, although it is critical for the PMHCNS to be proficient at this skill. There is often minimal difference between the curricula of the PMHCNS and PMHNP study programs. One might assume that the difference is in the clinical experience; however, this is not consistently or clearly specified. Some university settings have suspended admissions to their master's level PMHCNS (and other CNS) programs, referring interested applicants to pursue CNS education at the doctoral level of education in the form of the doctorate of nursing practice (DNP) programs.

THE PMHCNS AND THE CONSENSUS MODEL

Some may have thought that the Consensus Model was simply another white paper written with thoughts and aspirations of a professional body wanting a seat at the adult table. It is clear that many other professions have already realigned their professional

Table 1
A sample of 5 programs of study for the PMHCNS and NP

Educational Program	NP	CNS
The Ohio State University[7]	"Theoretical and evidence-based clinical knowledge that is essential for comprehensive primary care and specialty practice in a variety of settings"[7] "Diagnose and manage acute episodic and long-term illnesses and emphasize health promotion, illness prevention, and interprofessional collaboration"[7]	"Expert in diagnosis, treatment, remediation and alleviation of illnesses and to promote health within a specialty population"[7] "Provides highly specialized nursing care, serves as the clinical nursing expert for a unit or service line; and also implements the role for clinical coordinator, case manager, staff and patient educator and participant in research projects"[7]
University of California, San Francisco[8] Psychiatric/ Mental Health Nursing "Advanced practice psychiatric nurses provide comprehensive patient-centered mental health care to individuals, groups, and families across the lifespan. An advanced practice psychiatric nurse may function as a Clinical Nurse Specialist, Nurse Practitioner or, in some cases, both"[8]	"Primary mental health care services including biopsychosocial assessment and diagnosis of patients with mental illness. Treatment modalities include both medication and psychotherapeutic management"[8]	"Incorporates research, clinical leadership, education, consultation, and expert clinical practice. Expert PMHCNS practice includes provision of psychotherapy"[8]
Vanderbilt University	"Assess, diagnose, plan, implement, intervene, manage and evaluate holistic plans of care— including treatment with psychotropic medications; individual, group and family psychotherapy; crisis intervention; case management and consultation"[9]	No program offered
University of Pittsburgh	"Prepared as a principal provider of primary health care who manages the care of adult psychiatric clients in a variety of settings on both an episodic and continuous basis"[10]	"Care of patients with psychiatric or psychosocial issues, including the delivery of psychotherapy. Nurses are prepared to be therapists, consultants, mental health educators, case managers, and supervisors"[a,10]

(continued on next page)

Table 1 (continued)		
Educational Program	**NP**	**CNS**
Indiana University Advanced Practice Psychiatric Mental Health Nurse. The program prepares the student to sit for PMHCNS or PMHNP certification examination[11]	"Designed to prepare graduate students in the diagnosis, treatment, and prevention of mental illness. The program also prepares students in case management, professional leadership, and interdisciplinary collaboration across a wide range of health care settings"[11]	"Designed to prepare graduate students in the diagnosis, treatment, and prevention of mental illness. The program also prepares students in case management, professional leadership, and interdisciplinary collaboration across a wide range of health care settings"[11]

Data retrieved from the identified school of nursing's current Web site as specified in the reference list.
 Abbreviation: NP, nurse practitioner.
 [a] MSN program applications suspended as of June 2011 in favor of the doctorate of nursing practice program for CNS education.

degrees to include doctoral level for the clinical expert degrees, that is, doctor of psychology, doctor of pharmacy, doctor of audiology, and doctor of physical therapy. The Consensus Model recommendations are vaguely reminiscent of the 1985 entry into practice proposal that mandated a dramatic philosophic shift regarding basic nursing education.[12] The realization that the entry into practice proposition was never implemented and the divisiveness that has since haunted our profession for years after have been quite a dose to swallow. Years of hard work and discussion preceded its appearance, but every stakeholder group would not buy in, and there was ultimately enough dissent to stop the proposition from ever becoming a reality, no matter how noble the cause. The move to provide consistent definitions and points of entry into advanced nursing practice is ambitious and necessary to move advanced practice nursing forward in a deliberate and thoughtful manner.

The Consensus Model for APRN regulation (2008) provides comprehensive definitions for the CNS and the certified nurse practitioner (CNP) along with the minimal educational requirements necessary for certification and entry on licensure into advanced nursing practice. The Consensus Model defines the CNP as one prepared to deliver expert care to the individual or family system in his or her area of practice expertise. The CNS fulfills this care function for individuals and families in addition to working within systems mentoring, facilitating change and evidenced-based practice. In addition to participating in the generation and use of evidence in nursing science, the PMHCNS is a provider of expert clinical care, consultation services, staff and consumer education, and clinical leadership. The PMHCNS acts as a mentor to nurse generalists and beginning APRNs, and provides clinical supervision to members of health care teams. Yet these skills are not clearly reflected by the ANCC certification and, as the role is slated for retirement, these skills are in danger of being lost. Given the scope of the PMHCNS and its broad responsibilities in an increasingly complex and evolving health care environment, it is imperative that the skills and functions that the PMHCNS has brought to the mental health table not be lost as the PMHCNS certification is retired. Those expert clinical, organizational, and mentoring skills must be preserved.

For a newly educated APRN interested in providing psychiatric and mental health nursing care, the FPMHNP will become the certification credential for entry into advanced mental health nursing practice, because the PMHCNS and PMHNP retires in 2014.[13] Therefore, the generality of specialty-focused designations becomes apparent as the current population and specialty designations collapse into fewer numbers, and this collapse will accurately reflect on the generalist's entry into advanced practice.

Mind the Gaps

Although the Consensus Model for APRN regulation articulates the CNS role, the foundational educational requirement for advanced practice nurses offers only vague direction regarding the educational requirements for the CNS. This vagueness is frequently reflected in the master's level curricula, in which there is minimal difference between the CNS and nurse practitioner (NP) curricula. Given the broader scope of CNS practice and the need for specialty expertise, the American Association of Colleges of Nursing recommendation for advanced nursing practice preparation to be at the doctoral level and the shift in several nursing programs in moving their CNS programs to a doctoral level seems appropriate. The DNP offers the educational venue for advanced NPs in the role of CNS to gain specialized knowledge that extends beyond the direct focus of the NP on patient care. The DNP with a specialty in psychiatric and mental health nursing is the logical next step. Although work on the practice doctorate began years ago, and thoughtful development and discussion of purpose and curricula have since ensued, the PMHCNS needs to be at the table as these discussions continue.

Another difficulty in the current interpretation of the Consensus Model lies in the absence of statements that would directly address some critical elements of the PMHCNS (see **Table 1**). Apparent in this discovery is the notion that several roles of the PMHCNS do not consistently appear in writing within current curricula or within the ANCC certification requirements for roles incorporating psychiatric mental health care, even though these roles will undoubtedly continue to be practiced by those who retain the PMHCNS designation. The roles include education and mentoring of nurses who provide psychiatric and mental health care, clinical supervision, debriefing, facilitating system changes, supporting development and use of evidence-based approaches aimed at improving nursing care, promoting improved clinical outcomes for psychiatric and mental health patients and their families, facilitating ethical decision making, and promoting diversity.

MOVING FORWARD

The role of the PMHCNS is at a crossroads: evolution or extinction. Although advanced practice roles may be maintained, ranks are dwindling and the ANCC certification examination is slated to be retired in 2014. The future of the PMHCNS, for those certified before 2014, requires vigilance to continue educational development and clinical practice and to maintain the advanced practice nursing credential and role. After 2014, when the PMHCNS certification will no longer be available, the ranks, as currently defined through certification, will continue to dwindle by attrition. The current PMHCNS certification will thus become extinct; however, the role can survive. This is not the time for complacency. We are challenged to educate others on the role and to demonstrate the value that the PMHCNS brings to the patient, family, multidisciplinary team, organization, community, and profession. Nursing practice has evolved over the years to become the most available profession for the patient. The nurse is the professional who spends most time with the patient and family, who knows the intricacies of the family, who has connected with the family unit in a way that other health professionals have not had the opportunity to, and is truly able to provide holistic care to the individual and the family. The challenge for the PMHCNS is to clearly demonstrate and communicate the comprehensive role that incorporates the mental health care of patient and family systems as well as the nursing and health care systems. Knowledge of physical, psychological, and social systems, and how they interact, allows for unique patient views and world views that guide our practice.

As PMHCNSs, we need to mentor nurses in mental health areas as well as throughout patient care systems to address the psychiatric mental health needs of patients in whatever setting they present. The PMHCNS is the consultant to mental health nursing staff and nurses in other general and specialty areas regarding care of the individual with mental health issues and needs. While institutions of higher learning evolve curricula for the newly devised advanced practice professional, nursing needs to pledge not to give up roles within patient care that are best delivered by the PMHCNS. We need to be actively involved in development of the evolving DNP with a specialty in psychiatric mental health nursing, to ensure that nurses remain at the table with other mental health professionals, as credible skilled clinicians offering unique holistic views and able to create and use evidence to guide practice.

Although the title may be retained, the scope of practice is more important. We must not be content to wait for change to arrive. We must be an active part of the evolution that is occurring if our role is to survive. Drawing on the examples of the psychiatric nursing leaders who have paved the way, it is up to us to be actively involved in this changing world. With a broad scope of specialty practice, the PMHCNS is well suited to continue implementing this role. The PMHCNS has a voice and it must be used. We are challenged to explore, advise, and advocate as to how the unique qualities of the PMHCNS, which are in jeopardy of extinction, can be integrated into advanced practice psychiatric mental health nursing education and practice as it continues to develop. Looking toward the future, it is up to the PMHCNS to ensure that the ability to provide a variety of psychiatric and mental health treatment modalities is maintained, so that the advanced practice nurse can continue to address psychiatric and mental health needs holistically, across settings and across the health care continuum.

REFERENCES

1. APRN Joint Dialogue Group Report, 2008. Consensus Model for APRN regulation: licensure, accreditation, certification and education. Available at: www.aacn.nche.edu/Education/pdf/APRNReport.pdf. Accessed November 14, 2011.
2. American Nurses Credentialing Center (ANCC), 2011. Consensus Model for APRN regulations, frequently asked questions. Available at: http://www.nursecredentialing.org/APRN-FAQ.aspx. Accessed October 28, 2011.
3. Critchley DL, Maurin JT. The clinical nurse specialist in psychiatric mental health nursing. New York: John Wiley and Sons; 1985.
4. Peplau H. Specialization in professional nursing. Nurs Sci 1965;3:268.
5. American Nurses Credentialing Center (ANCC), 2010. 2009 Role delineation study: clinical nurse specialist in adult psychiatric and mental health nursing—national survey results. Available at: http://www.nursecredentialing.org/Documents/Certification/RDS/2009RDSSurveys/AdultPsychCNS-2009RDS.aspx. Accessed November 1, 2011.
6. American Nurses Credentialing Center (ANCC), 2010. 2010 ANCC certification statistics. Available at: http://www.nursecredentialing.org/Certification/FacultyEducators/Statistics.aspx. Accessed November 1, 2011.

7. The Ohio State University School of Nursing (OSU). Available at: http://nursing.osu.edu/Display.aspx?code=141. Accessed November 21, 2011.

8. University of California San Francisco School of Nursing (UCSF). Available at: http://nursing.ucsf.edu/programs/specialties/psychiatricmental-health-nursing. Accessed November 21, 2011.

9. Vanderbilt University School of Nursing (UV). Available at: http://www.nursing.vanderbilt.edu/msn/pmhnp_plan.html. Accessed November 21, 2011.

10. University of Pittsburgh: School of Nursing (UP). Available at: http://www.nursing.pitt.edu/academics/masters/clinical.jsp. Accessed November 21, 2011.

11. Indiana University School of Nursing. Available at: http://nursing.iupui.edu/. Accessed November 21, 2011.

12. Christy TE. A recurring issue in nursing history. Lippincott Williams & Wilkins. Am Jrl Nur 1980;80(3):485–8. Available at. http://www.jstor.org/stable/3469921. Accessed November 11, 2011.

13. American Nurse Credentialing Center APRN Corner: Frequently asked questions. 2012. Available at: http://www.nursecredentialing.org/Certification/APRNCorner/APRN-FAQ.aspx#17. Accessed March 16, 2012.

Indicators of Resilience in Family Members of Adults with Serious Mental Illness

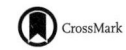

Jaclene A. Zauszniewski, PhD, RN-BC[a],*,
Abir K. Bekhet, PhD, RN, HSMI[b], M. Jane Suresky, DNP, PMHCNS-BC[a]

KEYWORDS

- Resilience • Family caregivers • Serious mental illness • Risk/vulnerability factors
- Positive/protective factors

KEY POINTS

- Resilient family members of persons with mental illness can overcome the stress and burden that may otherwise compromise their health and quality of life.
- Central constructs of resilience theory are risk/vulnerability factors, positive/protective factors, indicators of resilience, and outcomes of resilience.
- Seven indicators of resilience, including acceptance, hardiness, hope, mastery, self-efficacy, sense of coherence, and resourcefulness, have been studied in family members of persons with mental illness.

The most recent US census found that nearly 62 million adults had a diagnosed mental disorder and about 14 million were diagnosed with a serious mental illness.[1] Before deinstitutionalization and advances in the development of medications, persons with serious mental illnesses lived in institutions, apart from their families. Today, these individuals live in our communities. Although some adults with mental illness live independently, many live with family members, who care for them and help them manage daily activities.[2,3] Even if they are not in the same household, family members are generally involved in their care and support.[4] Family members of persons with serious mental illness may endure considerable stress and burden that can compromise their own health and quality of life and impair the functioning of the family. However, if family members are resilient, they can overcome stress associated with providing care for a loved one with a mental illness and preserve their own health and the health of their family.[5,6] This integrative review summarizes current research on resilience in adult family members who have a relative with a serious mental

This article is updated from its first appearance in Nurs Clin N Am 2010;45:613–26.
[a] Frances Payne Bolton School of Nursing, Case Western Reserve University, 2120 Cornell Road, Cleveland, OH 44106-4904, USA; [b] Marquette University College of Nursing, 530 North 16th Street, Milwaukee, WI 53233, USA
* Corresponding author.
E-mail address: jaz@case.edu

Psychiatr Clin N Am 38 (2015) 131–146
http://dx.doi.org/10.1016/j.psc.2014.11.009
0193-953X/15/$ – see front matter © 2015 Elsevier Inc. All rights reserved.

disorder, including major depressive disorder, bipolar disorder, schizophrenia, and panic disorder.[7] Although some studies have included children and young siblings providing care for a relative with a mental illness, this review focuses on family members who are adults.

RESILIENCE

Early writings on resilience came from researchers who focused on its development in children and adolescents.[8,9] More recently, there has been an increased interest in resilience in adults[10] and families.[11] The concept of resilience was described by Rutter[12(p119)] as "relative resistance to psychosocial risk experiences," and by Luthar and colleagues[13] as "a dynamic process encompassing positive adaptation within the context of significant adversity." Richardson[14(p308)] defined resilience as "the process of coping with adversity, change, or opportunity in a manner that results in the identification, fortification, and enrichment of resilient qualities or protective factors." Definitions of resilience in caregivers vary,[15] but they all share the characteristic of overcoming adversity to not only survive the day-to-day burden of caring for a family member who is mentally ill, but to thrive, that is, to grow into a stronger, yet more flexible and healthier person.[16] Resilience theory focuses on the strengths possessed by individuals or families that enable them to overcome adversity. The central constructs of resilience theory are risk or vulnerability factors, positive or protective factors, indicators of resilience, and outcomes of resilience.

RISK/VULNERABILITY FACTORS

Risk factors have been conceptualized as events or conditions associated with adversity or factors that reduce one's ability to resist stressors or overcome adversity.[10] Vulnerability factors include traits, genetic predispositions, or environmental and biological deficits.[10] Potential risk factors in caring for a family member with a serious mental illness include caregiver strain, feelings of stigma, client dependence, and family disruption; together, these factors can seriously compromise the caregiver's resilience.[17] **Table 1** lists examples of risk or vulnerability factors that were identified in studies of family members of adults with serious mental illness.

Having a family member with a mental illness in itself puts family members and the family unit at risk for experiencing negative outcome in terms of the physical and

Table 1
Risk/vulnerability factors, protective factors, and outcomes of resilience indicators identified in studies of family members of adults with mental illness

Risk/Vulnerability Factors	Protective/Positive Factors	Outcomes of Resilience Indicators
Family member with mental illness	Control appraisal[18]	Expressed emotion[31]
Lack of mental health services/support	Positive appraisal[25]	Psychological well-being[18,32]
Threat appraisal[18]	Personal religiosity[26]	Family adaptation[33]
Caregiver age[19,20]	Psychoeducation[27–29]	Family functioning[34,35]
Education[19,20]	Social support[19]	Knowledge and understanding[36–38]
Caregiver burden/stress[21–23]	Positive cognitions[17]	Morale[36]
Caregiver strain[23]	Length of time since diagnosis[20,30]	Satisfaction[39]
Family disruption[23]	Age of care recipient[30]	Relationship to mentally ill person[32]
Stressful life events[24]		Caregiver burden[19,24,39–41]
Avoidance coping[21]		Quality of life[20,22,23]

mental health of individual family members and the functioning of the family.[32,42] When the mentally ill family member is living in the same household, this may put relatives at greater risk for compromised health,[32,42] and the risk for poor health may increase even more when the mentally ill person requires ongoing supervision or direct personal care.[36] Finally, the lack of available, accessible, or affordable mental health services for families with a person with mental illness has been identified as a risk factor in several studies.[36]

Some demographic features of family caregivers may increase their vulnerability to compromised health, including age[19,20,26,39] and level of education.[19,20] The studies suggested that older family members and those who have less education may be more prone to health problems and disruptions in family functioning. Family caregivers who appraise their situation as threatening are thought to be at greater risk.[18] They may perceive caregiving as burdensome or stressful,[21–23] and they report greater feelings of strain,[23] more stressful life events,[24] and greater disruption in family functioning.[23] Perlick and colleagues[21] found a high use of avoidance coping strategies by family members of persons with mental illness. Although avoidance coping may be a less than optimal method for coping, it is possible that this coping method may also be protective; thus, risk factors in one context may be protective in another.[10,12,43]

PROTECTIVE/POSITIVE FACTORS

According to Rutter,[44] protective factors reduce the impact of risk, decrease negative reactions to risk, promote resilience, and create opportunities for family caregivers to include strategies for maintaining a positive success. Protective factors identified in studies of family members of adults with mental illness reflect their appraisal of the caregiving situation itself and their personal beliefs. A positive appraisal of the situation[18] and positive cognitions[17] have both been linked to greater resilience and better health outcomes. In addition, Murray-Swank and colleagues[26] found that personal religiosity helped family members of persons with mental illness adapt to the situation. Although positive appraisal, positive cognitions, and personal religiosity are intrapersonal factors that provide protection for family members of persons with mental illness, interpersonal and extrapersonal protective factors have also been identified. Social support[19,38] and psychoeducation programs for family members[27–29,38,45] have been found to have positive effects on resilience and health outcomes for individuals and the family unit. Also, the duration of the caregiving experience, which is closely tied to increasing age of the mentally ill care recipient, has been associated with resilience and quality of life in family members of adults with serious mental illness.[30]

RESILIENCE IN FAMILY CAREGIVERS

To date, 5 studies of resilience in family members of persons with mental illness have been published and 3 of them were conducted over a decade ago. Enns and colleagues[46] collected data on family resources, perceptions, and overall adaptation of 111 family members of adults admitted to a psychiatric hospital to identify factors that might contribute to resilience in family members. The data collected on major study variables were compared with averages on similar measures in the general population, and family members in the study were found to be similar to the general population on measures of health ($p\text{-}norms = .546$) and well-being ($p\text{-}norms = .018$), role performance ($p\text{-}norms = .103$), task accomplishment ($p\text{-}norms = .424$), and values and norms ($p\text{-}norms = .308$). They had significantly less perceived social support, esteem, and communication and were less likely to seek spiritual support than the general population. However, they were more likely to acquire social support and to mobilize the immediate family, and they had higher scores on affective expression, communication, and perceived control.

Marsh and colleagues[47] conducted a national survey to investigate the effects of resilience among family members of people with mental illness. The 131 family members in the sample were mothers, fathers, wives, husbands, sisters, brothers, daughters, sons, and extended family members. Family members were asked to identify strengths within themselves, their family, or their mentally ill family member that they thought were developed in relation to their family member's mental illness. Personal resilience was reported most frequently (by 99% of participants), followed by family resilience (88%) and resilience in the mentally ill family member (76%). Mannion,[48] who did a follow-up analysis of the data from that survey, found that most spouses (83%) described a process of adaptation and recovery and cited personal resilience as a major factor in facilitating positive changes. Personal resilience was described more strongly than family resilience or resilience in the mentally ill family member.

The aforementioned studies of resilience were all conducted in the 1990s. More recently, 2 studies examined resilience in family members of persons with serious mental illness. Herbert and colleagues[49] found that 24% of the offspring of parents with schizophrenia (n = 11) were highly resilient; 60% (n = 27) were classified in a middle range, and 15% (n = 7) were low in resilience. They also reported that those who were in the middle range and higher on resilience were also those offspring who reported more supportive relationships with their parent who had schizophrenia. Jain and Singh[50] conducted a study to determine whether family caregivers of persons with schizophrenia were similar to caregivers of persons with bipolar disorder in their resilience and perceived quality of life and whether their resilience was similarly associated with their perceived quality of life. The findings showed that resilience and its correlation with quality of life were the same for both groups of caregivers. However, other recent research has identified several strengths, characteristics, qualities, and virtues that are viewed as indicators of resilience,[5,14,16] including acceptance, hardiness, hope, mastery, self-efficacy, sense of coherence, and resourcefulness. Studies that examined these resilience indicators in family members of persons with mental illness are reviewed later.

Acceptance

Acceptance has been defined as a willingness to fully experience internal events, including thoughts, feelings, memories, and sensations.[51] It refers to an active process of understanding and having a sense of obligation and resignation to an unchangeable situation.[52] Christensen and Jacobson[53] defined acceptance as the ability to tolerate what one might regard as an unpleasant behavior of a relative with mental illness, with some understanding of the deeper meaning of that behavior and an appreciation of its value and importance. Six studies of family members of adults with mental illness have suggested that acceptance of the caregiving situation and the relative's diagnosis of mental illness is an indicator of resilience. In a study of 80 family members conducted in Ghana, Quinn[54] found that in rural areas, families were more accepting of the mental illness and therefore more supportive of their loved ones. Fortune and colleagues,[18] who examined relationships among perceptions of their loved one's psychosis, coping strategies, cognitive appraisals, and distress with 42 relatives of adults with schizophrenia in the United Kingdom, found that family members who expressed greater acceptance of their relative's psychosis, its severity, and consequences experienced less distress ($r = -0.66$, $P<.001$). In addition, acceptance, along with positive reframing and a lower tendency toward self-blame, was found to mediate the effects of perceptions of their relative's illness on their distress.

In 3 international qualitative studies of family members of persons with serious mental illness, acceptance emerged as a major theme. In a study conducted in Thailand by Sethabouppha and Kane,[52] 17 Buddhist family members of persons with mental illness shared their beliefs and perspectives on their experiences with their mentally ill family member. The themes they identified included management, compassion, and acceptance. Mizuno and colleagues[55] studied the caregiving experiences of 12 husbands whose spouses had schizophrenia in Japan. The content analysis revealed 6 major themes, the first of which was the identification and acceptance of the mental disorder. Radfar and colleagues[56] described experiences of 26 family members of persons suffering from depression in Iran. From their content emerged a main theme they called "turbulent life," which had 5 subcomponents, one of which was a delay in acceptance of their family member's depression.

Only one study has examined the needs of caregivers of people with mental illness in the United States. This intervention study by Eisner and Johnson[31] examined the effects of a psychoeducation program for 28 families who had a family member diagnosed with bipolar disorder. Their intervention also taught acceptance to the family members to decrease their anger and minimize self-blame. One week after intervention, the family members were found to have more knowledge about their relative's illness, but their anger and self-blame remained unchanged. However, the results cannot be generalized because of the small sample size, and because baseline scores on criticism and anger were low. Furthermore, the study used self-report measures and the length of the period was only a week, making it difficult to practice or implement what had been learned. Despite its limitations, this intervention study did address the needs of family members of persons with mental illness. However, more intervention studies are needed.

Hardiness

Hardiness was defined by Kobasa[57] as a personality characteristic comprising 3 interrelated concepts: control, commitment, and challenge. However, others have said that hardiness involves cognitive and behavioral flexibility, motivation to follow through with plans, and endurance when faced with adversity.[58] In caregivers, hardiness has been found to minimize the burden of caregiving,[59] enable caregivers to appraise the caregiving situation more positively,[60] and use problem-focused coping methods, including help-seeking strategies.[61]

Two studies have examined hardiness in family members of persons with mental illness. Greef and colleagues[33] studied 30 families of mentally ill young adults (average age of 24 years) in Belgium, most of whom were diagnosed with schizophrenia or other psychosis or mood or anxiety disorder. Of 12 potential resilience indicators examined in that study, hardiness was found to have the strongest correlation with family adaptation ($r = 0.63$; $P<.01$). Also, Han and colleagues,[34] who collected data from 365 Korean families providing care for a relative with a chronic mental illness, found a significant correlation between hardiness and family functioning ($r = 0.51$, $P<.001$). Neither of the 2 studies examined interventions; clearly intervention studies are needed to test the effects of programs to improve functioning in families with a relative with chronic mental illness. Large representative samples are also needed as well as more focused homogeneous samples in terms of type of mental illness, length of illness, and age of the mentally ill person to be able to generalize the findings.

Mastery

Mastery has been defined as the extent to which individuals believe they have control over what happens in their life.[62] Thus, it can be conceptualized as a dimension of coping with stress that reflects a sense of personal control over potentially adverse circumstances. A sense of mastery has been identified as a resource that may facilitate family adaptation to mental illness.[63] In family caregivers, greater mastery has been associated with lower caregiver burden and psychological distress and a greater sense of competence in the caregiving role.[21,64]

Five studies of family members of persons with mental illness have examined mastery, which may be viewed as an indicator of resilience. Murray-Swank and colleagues[26] studied 83 caregivers of persons with serious mental illness to examine whether religiosity was associated with psychosocial adjustment and caregiver burden. The findings indicated that younger age and greater religiosity were both associated with mastery ($r = -0.28$, $P = .009$, and $r = 0.26$, $P = .017$). Perlick and colleagues[21] studied 500 caregivers of adults with bipolar disorder to identify caregivers at risk for poor health in relation to caregiving and stress. The caregivers comprised 3 groups: those who were considered "burdened," those who were considered "effective," and those who were considered "stigmatized." Those who were "burdened" experienced poorer health outcomes than the other 2 groups. They also reported lower mastery than the other groups ($F [1, 2] = 47.97$, $P<.001$).

Lau and Pang,[25] who examined how 129 relatives providing care for persons with major psychiatric illnesses appraised their caregiving, found that a better sense of mastery was associated with less negative appraisal ($r = -0.24$, $P = .03$); however, no relationship was found between mastery and positive appraisal of caregiving itself. Rose and colleagues[64] evaluated feelings of burden and sense of mastery of 30 family members of relatives with mental illness. No significant association was found between caregiver burden and mastery. The researchers explained that the lack of significance may have resulted from the mastery scale's inability to capture perceived lack of control among family members.

Pollio and colleagues[29] compared the effects of a psychoeducation group for 9 family members of adults with mental illness to usual services for family members. The 7 family members who completed the intervention showed significant improvements on 4 of 5 items measuring knowledge and mastery, and on the specific item that reflected feeling in control, scores increased, although not significantly. Although these findings should be interpreted with caution, given the small sample, the results suggest that psychoeducation enhances a sense of mastery among family caregivers of persons with mental disorders. Future intervention research should use larger samples and analytical models with behavioral measures for both families and their ill members. Furthermore, outcomes should be measured immediately after the intervention, and 3 months, 6 months, and 1-year after intervention to indicate whether mastery can be maintained over time.

Hope

Hope has been characterized as multidimensional and dynamic, with elements of confidence yet uncertain expectation of a positive outcome.[65] Hope is created from memories and influenced by relationships with others; it promotes forward movement and provides new insights and a sense of purpose.[66] Hope has been identified as an integral part of family members' ability to cope with mental illness in a family member.[67] Nine studies have examined hope or optimism in family members of adults with mental illness. Four studies were qualitative; one study quantitatively examined associations, and 4 studies were intervention studies. Bland and Darlington,[67] who conducted in-depth qualitative interviews with 16 family members in Australia to explore the meaning and importance of hope, found that hopefulness was an integral part of the coping process used by the family members. Karp and Tanarugsachock[68] conducted in-depth qualitative interviews with 50 family members of adults with depression, bipolar disorder, or schizophrenia to explore how family members managed their emotions over the course of the family member's mental illness. They found that it was at the point of diagnosis that feelings of hope were provoked in family members.

Using individual interviews and focus groups, Stjernswärd and Ostman[42] explored the experiences of 18 family members living with an individual with depression. The family members described hope as a motivating force for finding effective treatment, a trustworthy physician, a meaningful and productive future, and improved quality of life for both the mentally ill family member and themselves. Tweedell and colleagues[69] studied the experiences of 8 family members with a chronically mentally ill relative. During interviews conducted 5 times over a 1-year period, family members described hopes and fears associated with interpersonal relationships with their family member. They were unanimous in hoping their relatives would gain relief from suffering psychotic symptoms, return to their former selves, be independent in caring for themselves, and live a worthwhile and productive life. They also expressed cautious optimism that treatment would last, and some worried about losing hope for treatment, symptom management, and improved quality of life for their family member.

Hernandez and colleagues[40] examined hope and family burden among 54 Latino families of individuals with schizophrenia. Hierarchical linear regression analyses revealed an increase in hope in family members of persons with severe mental illness that was associated with decreased caregiver burden and exceeded the effects explained by the diagnosed person's length of illness and severity of symptoms. Redlich and colleagues[70] tested an intervention that teaches communication strategies and uses a mediated learning approach aimed to positively alter cognitions in family members who have a relative with a serious mental illness. The findings indicated that family members who received the intervention had significant increases in hope in comparison with the control group. Pickett-Schenk and colleagues[36] studied 424 families of persons with schizophrenia who took part in an intervention designed to instill hope by providing education and support. Data were collected before the intervention and at 3 and 6 months following the program. At 3 months after intervention, greater satisfaction with the education and support components of the intervention program predicted increased knowledge of the causes and treatment of mental illness ($\beta = 0.29$, $P<.001$ and $\beta = 0.21$, $P<.001$), greater understanding of mental health services ($\beta = 0.25$, $P<.001$ and $\beta = 0.34$, $P<.001$), and improved morale ($\beta = 0.19$, $P<.001$ and $\beta = 0.18$, $P<.001$). Some effects of satisfaction persisted at 6 months, but the effects on morale and understanding of mental health services were not found at 6 months after intervention.

Pickett-Schenk and colleagues[32] also examined the effectiveness of the same intervention for 462 family members of adults with schizophrenia. As in the previous study, the intervention included education about the causes and treatment of mental illness, problem-solving and communication skills training, and family support. Outcomes were evaluated before intervention and at 3 and 6 months after intervention. Family members in the intervention group reported better psychological well-being than those in a wait-list control group, as indicated by fewer depressive symptoms ($\beta = -1.64$, $P = .04$), greater emotional role functioning ($\beta = 5.69$, $P = .03$) and vitality

($\beta = 3.57, P = .04$), and less negative views toward relationships with their mentally ill family member ($\beta = -0.73$, $P<.01$). These effects were maintained over time.

In a follow-up study, Pickett-Schenk and colleagues[37] examined the effects of the same intervention on family members' knowledge of causes and treatment of schizophrenia, problem-solving skills, and need for information. Those in the intervention group reported greater gains in knowledge than a waiting list control group ($\beta = 0.84$, $P<.01$), fewer needs for information on coping with positive and negative symptoms of their family member's illness ($\beta = -0.63$, $P<.05$ and $\beta = -0.80$, $P<.001$, respectively), and greater gains in problem management ($\beta = -1.00$, $P<.001$), basic facts about mental illness and its treatment ($\beta = -0.73$, $P<.01$), and community resources ($\beta = -0.07$, $P<.05$). The effects were maintained over time. Of these 4 intervention studies focused on increasing hope, one was a pilot study[70] and one was a randomized controlled trial,[32] which had some limitations, including a possible placebo effect and use of self-reported data, making it difficult to determine whether the intervention brought about actual improvements in the family members' relationships with their mentally ill relatives.[32] Intervention studies that include behavioral observations rather than self-report are needed.

Self-Efficacy

Self-efficacy refers to an individual's confidence in dealing with challenging and stressful encounters,[71] or one's self-evaluation of one's capacity for performing an activity or task to achieve a specific goal.[72] In family caregivers of persons with mental illness, greater self-efficacy has been linked with better management of behavioral problems in care receivers, less perceived stress, and lower subjective burden.[5] Four studies have examined self-efficacy of family members of adults with mental illness; 3 of the studies involved relatives of persons with schizophrenia, and none were conducted in the United States. In a correlational study of 62 family members of persons with schizophrenia conducted in Turkey, Durmaz and Okanli[41] investigated the association between self-efficacy and caregiver burden and reported a significant inverse relationship that indicated that greater self-efficacy was associated with lower caregiver burden.

Two studies involved Chinese family members of persons with schizophrenia. Cheng and Chan[28] evaluated the effectiveness of a psychoeducation program with 64 family caregivers recruited from a mental hospital in Hong Kong. Those in the psychoeducation group improved more in self-efficacy than a group receiving routine care ($t = -7.16$, $P<.01$). The effectiveness of the psychoeducation program was then tested in a second study by Chan and colleagues[27] with 73 Chinese family members of persons with schizophrenia; this study also examined longer-term effects. Postintervention effects on self-efficacy were similar to those in the first study. The effects were sustained at 6 months, but not at 12 months, suggesting a need for continued intervention to promote self-efficacy.

The fourth study was conducted in Sweden by Ali and colleagues,[45] and it consisted of 241 family members of persons with mental illness; the diagnosis was unspecified. The study was an intervention trial to compare Web-based support to providing educational/informational materials in a folder on outcomes that included stress, self-efficacy, well-being, health, and quality of life. The findings showed that those who received the folder with educational information had lower stress, greater self-efficacy, and better health and quality of life than those in the Web-based intervention group; however, those in the Web-based group improved more in well-being than those in the educational information folder group. Although these studies provided promising results, they had several limitations. For example, the measures used were self-reported, and the mentally ill persons were mostly men, whereas caregivers were mostly women.[27,28,45] Finally, the studies included only family members who were willing to participate, and this group could have already had more motivation to change, leading to positive outcomes.[27,28,45]

Sense of Coherence

A sense of coherence has been defined as a global orientation toward life that involves cognitive, behavioral, and motivational elements and is expressed in the belief that the world is comprehensible, manageable, and meaningful.[73] Family sense of coherence refers to the belief of family members that the internal and external environment is structured and predictable and resources are available; they perceive life and their situation as a meaningful challenge and consider that they can exert an influence on the course of events.[33] Nine studies have evaluated a sense of coherence in family members of adults with mental illness; 6 of them were international studies. Han and colleagues,[34] who examined the influence of a sense of coherence on family functioning in 365 Korean families providing care for a relative with a chronic mental illness, found a significant positive correlation between sense of coherence and family functioning ($r = 0.43$; $P<.001$). Similar findings were reported in a recent US study by Suresky and colleagues,[35] who reported that a greater sense of coherence was associated with lower family disruption ($r = -0.37$; $P = .03$). However, they also found that sense of coherence did not mediate the effects of strain on family disruption.

In a study of 556 Thai family caregivers of adults with schizophrenia, Pipatananond and colleagues[19] found that sense of coherence was influenced by education ($\gamma = 0.29$, $P<.001$), income ($\gamma = 0.28$, $P<.001$), social support ($\gamma = 0.20$, $P<.001$), and perceived seriousness of illness ($\gamma = 0.23$, $P<.001$), and sense of coherence had a direct negative effect on caregiver burden ($\beta = 0.16$, $P<.001$).[19] In a study of 243 Taiwanese family caregivers of a relative with schizophrenia, Hsiao and Tsai[39] reported that female gender, greater family demands, and lower sense of coherence were associated with caregiver burden, whereas caregiver satisfaction was positively associated with older age and higher sense of coherence. Thus, with the exception of sense of coherence, correlates of caregiver burden seemed to be somewhat distinct from those of caregiver satisfaction.

In a study of 226 relatives of persons with severe mental illness, Weimand and colleagues[74] found women, particularly those who were single, widowed, or divorced, reported greater caregiver burden. They also found that relatives who reported greater caregiver burden also reported poorer health, and both caregiver burden and poor health were associated with lower sense of coherence. Mizuno and colleagues[20] investigated sense of coherence and quality of life of 34 Japanese caregivers of persons with schizophrenia. They reported that sense of coherence was found to be influenced by the family caregivers' age, educational level, duration of illness, and whether they lived with the diagnosed individual. The findings also showed a significant correlation between sense of coherence and quality of life.

In a study of 60 American women family members of adults with serious mental illness, Suresky and colleagues[22] found that caregiver burden had a negative effect on sense of coherence ($\beta = -0.33$; $P<.01$), whereas sense of coherence accounted for 41% of the variance in quality of life and partially mediated the effects of caregiver burden on quality of life.[22] In a follow-up study on the same women, Zauszniewski and colleagues[17] found that the effects of caregiver burden on sense of coherence were mediated by positive cognitions, which served as protective factors. Finally, Greef and colleagues[33] examined sense of coherence as an indicator of adaptation in 30 families of mentally ill persons in Belgium. Hardiness showed the strongest correlation with sense of coherence ($r = 0.63$; $P<.01$).

In Sweden, Jonsson and colleagues[38] tested a 10-session educational invention with 34 family members of persons with bipolar disorder. The findings revealed that bipolar disorder had a significant negative impact on family members, but the educational intervention facilitated their understanding of the condition and ability to manage their stress. Sense of coherence increased over time, but not significantly, which is consistent with Antonovsky's conceptualization of sense of coherence as a relative constant throughout life.[73] Thus, only one intervention study was found whereby a sense of coherence was measured as an outcome, although the intervention itself was not focused directly on enhancing the sense of coherence. The other studies reviewed had some limitations. Most were either cross-sectional[19,20,33,34,74] or secondary analyses,[17,22,35] and therefore, it is difficult to assess changes in study variables over time. Furthermore, convenience sampling limits the generalizability of the findings, and the samples were heterogeneous in type of mental illness, length of illness, single parent or intact family, and age of the mentally ill family member.[33] Finally, given the small samples, caution must be used in drawing conclusions from the findings.[17,22,33]

Resourcefulness

Resourcefulness may be defined as cognitive and behavioral skills that are used to prevent potentially negative effects of thoughts, feelings, or sensations on the performance of daily activities[75] and to obtain assistance from others when unable to function independently.[76] Personal and social resourcefulness skills are complementary, can fluctuate over time, and are equally important for optimal quality of life.[77] Five studies have examined resourcefulness in family caregivers of persons with serious mental illness. Wang and colleagues[24] examined the effects of resourcefulness on stressful life events, psychiatric care activities, and the burden faced by 81 family caregivers of schizophrenic adolescents. The study found that 24.5% of the variance ($F [5, 75] = 6.20$, $P<.001$) in caregiver burden was explained by psychiatric care activities and the interaction of stressful life events and resourcefulness, indicating that resourcefulness moderated the adverse effects of stressful life events on caregiver burden.

Zauszniewski and colleagues[30] studied 60 women family members of adults diagnosed with schizophrenia, bipolar disorder, depression, or a panic anxiety disorder to identify factors that might affect family members' resourcefulness. Increasing age of the mentally ill person and longer time since diagnosis were associated with greater personal resourcefulness ($r = 0.32$, $P<.01$ and $r = 0.35$, $P<.01$, respectively). The women caregivers of adults with schizophrenia had greater personal resourcefulness ($t [1, 52] = 4.19$, $P<.01$ and $t [1, 52] = 2.62$, $P<.01$, respectively) than women who had a family member with bipolar disorder. Sisters of mentally ill persons reported more social resourcefulness than did mothers, daughters, or wives ($F [2, 59] = -3.16$, $P<.05$), but there were no significant differences in personal resourcefulness.

In a follow-up study of the same women, Zauszniewski and colleagues[23] found that African American and Caucasian women reported similar resourcefulness skills. However, in African Americans, greater caregiver burden was associated with lower resourcefulness ($r = -0.38$, $P<.0010$), and lower resourcefulness correlated with poorer mental health ($r = 0.53$, $P<.001$), suggesting that resourcefulness may mediate the adverse effects of caregiver burden on mental health. Another follow-up study by Zauszniewski and colleagues[17] focused on the mediating role played by positive cognitions, conceptualized as a protective factor on the relationship between caregiver burden and resourcefulness. The findings from that study provide support for resilience theory in that positive cognitions mediated the effects of caregiver burden on resourcefulness, an indicator of resilience. In a third follow-up study, conducted by Suresky and colleagues,[35] the relationship between resourcefulness and family disruption was examined in the women family members of persons with serious mental illness. Greater family disruption was found to be significantly associated with a lower resourcefulness in the women but not found to mediate the effects of caregiver strain on family disruption. All 5 of these studies were cross-sectional or secondary analyses, and none included an intervention. The studies also had some limitations, such as convenience samples, cross-sectional design, and small sample sizes.[17,23,30,35] Longitudinal studies of larger and more diverse samples of family members of mentally ill persons, including men, and persons from racial/ethnic minorities, are recommended. Intervention studies that teach cognitive behavioral self-help and help-seeking skills are also needed. Addressing the needs of family members of adolescents with serious mental illness is important; thus, intervention studies are needed for this vulnerable population.

OUTCOMES OF RESILIENCE

Resilience and resilience indicators have been linked with several positive health outcomes for individuals and families.[16] In the studies of family members of adults with mental illness included in this review, resilience indicators were found to be associated with, and, in some cases, to affect or predict outcomes indicative of mental and physical health and quality of life in individual family members and optimal family functioning. On the individual level, resilience indicators have been linked with decreased caregiver burden in family members of persons with mental illness.[19,24,39–41] In addition, decreased levels of expressed emotion, defined as a critical, hostile, or overinvolved attitude toward a relative with mental illness, have been associated with greater resilience in family members of persons with mental illness.[31] Other outcomes of resilience indicators found in studies of family members include better morale,[36] better satisfaction,[39] greater psychological well-being,[18,32] and improved knowledge and understanding of their family member's diagnosis.[36–38] Finally, 3 studies of family members found that enhanced quality of life was associated with indicators of resilience.[20,22,23] Greater resilience may also be linked with improvement in family members' relationships with their relative with a psychiatric diagnosis.[32] Finally, indicators of resilience have been associated with greater family adaptation and improvement in family functioning.[33–35]

SUMMARY

Although resilience has been examined in studies of family caregivers, including family members of persons with autism[78] and family members of persons with dementia,[79] few studies have included family members of persons with serious mental illness.[80] However, many researchers have examined characteristics of family members of persons with mental illness that may be considered indicators of resilience, including acceptance, hardiness, hope, mastery, self-efficacy, sense of coherence, and resourcefulness.[16] The research has consistently shown that family members who possess these positive characteristics are better able to manage and overcome adversity associated with caring for a family member diagnosed with a mental illness. Thus, enhancement of the resilience of family members of persons with serious mental illness will contribute to both their own well-being and the well-being of those for whom they provide care.

The findings from the studies reviewed here provide beginning evidence of the importance of focusing interventions on supporting and enhancing the resilience of family members of individuals with mental illness. However, additional studies to develop and test interventions for enhancing the characteristics constituting resilience in these family members are needed. Longitudinal studies that measure outcomes immediately after the intervention and at 3 months, 6 months, and 1 year after intervention would provide a picture of how resilience indicators can be enhanced and maintained over time. Also, more intervention studies that include behavioral observation rather than relying solely on self-report are needed. The evidence that emerges from testing well-developed interventions can inform clinical practice and enrich mental health professionals' ability to provide quality care for patients and their families.

Mental health professionals need to take a focused family therapy approach to manage stress and disruption in the family environment, to build the family's resilience and contribute to improvement in quality of life for the family and the mentally ill person. Assessing indicators of resilience in family members using standardized measures at the start of a treatment plan for family therapy could provide baseline data and direction for therapy. Assisting the family to gain knowledge of the mental illness and associated behaviors would facilitate understanding of the diagnosed family member's situation. In addition to using a cognitive approach to therapy, mental health professionals might suggest adjunct therapies for individual family members. Yoga, for example, has been found beneficial in reducing anxiety and depression; biofeedback is used to treat stress, and self-hypnosis provides a feeling of letting go of internal pressure and discomfort. At the conclusion of therapy, indicators of resilience should be measured again and compared with baseline results to provide further direction for therapy.

The information derived from the current review can be used by mental health professionals to plan primary, secondary, and tertiary prevention strategies to help caregivers of persons with mental illness regain, attain, or maintain optimal wellness. Assessing an individual's attitude toward mental illness, and his or her strengths and concerns, is vital to facilitate adjustment. Secondary prevention should be implemented when stress symptoms have already developed and should encompass interventions to increase resilience for those with stress as a result of their caregiving. Finally, tertiary prevention would help caregivers to use all existing internal and external resources to prevent further stress and maintain optimal wellness.

REFERENCES

1. National Institutes of Health, National Institute of Mental Health. (n.d.). Statistics: Any Disorder among Adults. Available at: http://www.nimh.nih.gov/statistics/1ANYDIS_ADULT.shtml. Accessed November 5, 2014.
2. Kohn-Wood LP, Wilson MN. The context of caretaking in rural areas: family factors influencing the level of functioning of seriously mentally ill patients living at home. Am J Community Psychol 2005;36(1/2):1–13.
3. Wynaden D, Ladzinski U, Lapsley J, et al. The caregiving experience: how much do health professionals understand? Collegian 2006;13(3):6–10.
4. Lively S, Friedrich RM, Rubenstein L. The effect of disturbing illness behaviors on siblings of persons with schizophrenia. J Am Psychiatr Nurses Assoc 2004;10(5): 222–32.
5. Saunders JC. Families living with severe mental illness: a literature review. Issues Ment Health Nurs 2003;24(2):175–98.

6. Walton-Moss B, Gerson L, Rose L. Effects of mental illness on family quality of life. Issues Ment Health Nurs 2005;26:627–42.
7. Bye L, Partridge J. State level classification of serious mental illness: a case for a more uniform standard. J Health Soc Policy 2004;19(2):1–29.
8. Garmezy N, Rutter M. Stress, coping, and development in children. New York: McGraw-Hill Book Company; 1983.
9. Werner EE, Smith RS. Overcoming the odds: high risk children from birth to adulthood. Ithaca (NY): Cornell University Press; 1992.
10. Smith-Osborne A. Life span and resiliency theory: a critical review. Adv Soc Work 2007;18(1):152–68.
11. McCubbin MA, McCubbin HI. Resiliency in families: a conceptual model of family adjustment and adaptation in response to stress and crises. In: McCubbin HI, Thompson AI, McCubbin MA, editors. Family assessment: resiliency, coping, and adaptation—Inventories for research and practice. Madison (WI): University of Wisconsin System; 1996. p. 1–64.
12. Rutter M. Resilience concepts and findings: implications for family therapy. J Fam Ther 1999;2:119–44.
13. Luthar S, Cicchetti D, Becker B. The construct of resilience: a critical evaluation and guidelines for future work. Child Dev 2000;71:543–62.
14. Richardson GE. The metatheory of resilience and resiliency. J Clin Psychol 2002; 58(3):307–21.
15. Gillespie BM, Chaboyer W, Wallis M. Development of a theoretically derived model of resilience through concept analysis. Contemp Nurse 2007;25(1/2):124–35.
16. Van Breda AD. Resilience theory: a literature review. Pretoria (South Africa): South African Military Health Service; 2001.
17. Zauszniewski JA, Bekhet AK, Suresky MJ. Effects on resilience of women family caregivers of adults with serious mental illness: the role of positive cognitions. Arch Psychiatr Nurs 2009;23(6):412–22.
18. Fortune DG, Smith JV, Garvey K. Perceptions of psychosis, coping, appraisals, and psychological distress in the relatives of patients with schizophrenia: an exploration using self-regulation theory. Br J Clin Psychol 2005;44:319–31.
19. Pipatananond P, Boontong T, Hanucharurnkul S, et al. Caregiver burden predictive model: an empirical test among caregivers for the schizophrenic. Thai J Nurs Res 2006;6(2):24–40.
20. Mizuno E, Iwasaki M, Sakai I. Sense of coherence and quality of life in family caregivers of persons with schizophrenia living in the community. Arch Psychiatr Nurs 2012;26(4):295–306.
21. Perlick DA, Rosenheck RA, Miklowitz DJ, et al. Caregiver burden and health in bipolar disorder: a cluster analytic approach. J Nerv Ment Dis 2008;196(6): 484–91.
22. Suresky MJ, Zauszniewski JA, Bekhet AK. Sense of coherence and quality of life in women family members of the seriously mentally ill. Issues Ment Health Nurs 2008;29:265–78.
23. Zauszniewski JA, Bekhet AK, Suresky MJ. Relationships among stress, depressive cognitions, resourcefulness and quality of life in female relatives of seriously mentally ill adults. Issues Ment Health Nurs 2009;30:142–50.
24. Wang S, Rong J, Chen C, et al. A study of stress, learned resourcefulness and caregiver burden among primary caregivers of schizophrenic adolescents. J Nurs (China) 2007;54(5):37–47.
25. Lau D, Pang A. Caregiving experience for Chinese caregivers of persons suffering from severe mental disorders. Hong Kong J Psychiatr 2007;17:75–80.

26. Murray-Swank AB, Lucksted A, Medoff DR, et al. Religiosity, psychosocial adjustment, and subjective burden of persons who care for those with mental illness. Psychiatr Serv 2006;57(3):361–5.
27. Chan SW, Yip B, Tso S, et al. Evaluation of a psychoeducation program from Chinese clients with schizophrenia and their family caregivers. Patient Educ Couns 2009;75:67–76.
28. Cheng LY, Chan SW. Psychoeducation program for Chinese family carers of members with schizophrenia. West J Nurs Res 2005;27(5):583–99.
29. Pollio DE, North CS, Osborne VA. Family-responsive psychoeducation groups for families with an adult member with mental illness: pilot results. Community Ment Health J 2002;38(5):413–21.
30. Zauszniewski JA, Bekhet AK, Suresky MJ. Factors associated with perceived burden, resourcefulness, and quality of life in female family members of adults with serious mental illness. J Am Psychiatr Nurses Assoc 2008;14(2): 125–35.
31. Eisner LR, Johnson SL. An acceptance-based psychoeducation intervention to reduce expressed emotion in relatives of bipolar patients. Behav Ther 2008;39: 375–85.
32. Pickett-Schenk SA, Cook JA, Steigman P, et al. Psychological well-being and relationship outcomes in a randomized study of family-led education. Arch Gen Psychiatry 2006;63:1043–50.
33. Greef AP, Vansteenwegen A, Ide M. Resiliency in families with a member with a psychological disorder. Am J Fam Ther 2006;34:285–300.
34. Han K, Lee P, Park E, et al. Family functioning and mental illness: a Korean correlational study. Asian J Nurs 2007;10(2):129–36.
35. Suresky MJ, Zauszniewski JA, Bekhet AK. Factors affecting disruption in families of adults with mental illness. Perspect Psychiatr Care 2014;50(4):235–42.
36. Pickett-Schenk SA, Cook JA, Laris A. Journey of Hope program outcomes. Community Ment Health J 2000;36:413–24.
37. Pickett-Schenk SA, Lippincott RC, Bennett C, et al. Improving knowledge about mental illness through family-led education: the journey of hope. Psychiatr Serv 2008;59(1):49–56.
38. Jonsson PD, Wijk H, Danielson E, et al. Outcomes of an educational intervention for the family of a person with bipolar disorder: a 2-year follow-up study. J Psychiatr Ment Health Nurs 2011;18:333–41.
39. Hsiao CY, Tsai YF. Caregiver burden and satisfaction in families of individuals with schizophrenia. Nurs Res 2014;63(4):260–9.
40. Hernandez M, Barrio C, Yamada AM. Hope and burden among Latino families of adults with schizophrenia. Fam Process 2013;52:697–708.
41. Durmaz H, Okanli A. Investigation of the effect of self-efficacy levels of caregiver family members of individuals with schizophrenia on burden of care. Arch Psychiatr Nurs 2004;28:290–4.
42. Stjernswärd S, Ostman M. Whose life am I living? Relatives living in the shadow of depression. Int J Soc Psychiatry 2008;54(4):358–69.
43. Ungar M. A constructionist discourse on resilience: multiple contexts, multiple realities among at-risk children and youth. Youth & Society 2004;35(3):341–65.
44. Rutter M. Psychosocial resilience and protective mechanisms. Am J Orthop 1987;57:316–31.
45. Ali L, Krevers B, Sjostrom N, et al. Effectiveness of web-based versus support interventions for young informal carers of persons with mental illness: a randomized controlled trial. Patient Educ Couns 2014;94:362–71.

46. Enns R, Reddon J, McDonald L. Indications of resilience among family members of people admitted to a psychiatric facility. Psychiatr Rehabil J 1999;23(2):127–33.
47. Marsh DT, Lefley HP, Evans-Rhodes D, et al. The family experience of mental illness: evidence for resilience. Psychiatr Rehabil J 1996;20(2):3–12.
48. Mannion E. Resilience and burden in spouses of people with mental illness. Psychiatr Rehabil J 1996;20(2):13–23.
49. Herbert HS, Manjula M, Philip M. Growing up with a parent having schizophrenia: experiences and resilience in the offspring. Indian J Psychol Med 2013;35(2):148–53.
50. Jain A, Singh DC. Resilience and quality of life in caregivers of schizophrenia and bipolar disorder patients. Global J Hum-Soc Science: Arts & Humanities – Psychology 2014;14(5):1–5.
51. Orsillo SM, Roemer L, Block-Lerner J, et al. Acceptance, mindfulness, and cognitive-behavioral therapy: comparisons, contrasts and applications to anxiety. In: Hayes SC, Follette VM, Linehan MM, editors. Mindfulness and acceptance: expanding the cognitive-behavioral tradition. New York: Guilford Press; 2004. p. 66–95.
52. Sethabouppha H, Kane C. Caring for the seriously mentally ill in Thailand: Buddhist family caregiving. Arch Psychiatr Nurs 2005;19(2):44–57.
53. Christensen A, Jacobson NS. Reconcilable differences. New York: Guilford Press; 2000.
54. Quinn N. Beliefs and community responses to mental illness in Ghana: the experiences of family carers. Int J Soc Psychiatry 2007;53(2):175–88.
55. Mizuno E, Iwasaki M, Sakai I. Subjective experiences of husbands of spouses with schizophrenia: an analysis of the husband's descriptions of their experiences. Arch Psychiatr Nurs 2011;25(5):366–75.
56. Radfar M, Ahmadi F, Fallahi khoshknab M. Turbulent life: the experiences of the family members of patients suffering from depression. J Psychiatr Ment Health Nurs 2014;21:249–56.
57. Kobasa SC. Stressful life events, personality and health: an inquiry into hardiness. J Pers Soc Psychol 1979;37:1–11.
58. Maddi SR. On hardiness and other pathways to resilience. Am Psychol 2005; 60(3):261–2.
59. DiBartolo M. Exploring self-efficacy and hardiness in spousal caregivers of individuals with dementia. J Gerontol Nurs 2002;28(4):24–33.
60. DiBartolo M, Soeken K. Appraisal, coping, hardiness, and self-perceived health in community-dwelling spouse caregivers of persons with dementia. Res Nurs Health 2003;26(6):445–58.
61. Clark P. Effects of individual and family hardiness on caregiver depression and fatigue. Res Nurs Health 2002;25(1):37–48.
62. Pearlin LI, Schooler C. The structure of coping. J Health Soc Behav 1978;19:2–21.
63. Rungreangkulkij S, Gillis CL. Conceptual approached to studying family caregiving for persons with severe mental illness. J Fam Nurs 2000;6(4):341–66.
64. Rose LE, Mallinson RK, Gerson LD. Mastery, burden, and areas of concern among family caregivers of mentally ill persons. Arch Psychiatr Nurs 2006; 20(1):41–51.
65. Dufault K, Martocchio B. Hope: its spheres and dimensions. Nurs Clin North Am 1985;20(2):379–91.
66. Parse RR. Hope: an international human becoming perspective. Boston (MA): Jones and Hartlett Publishers; 2000.
67. Bland R, Darlington Y. The nature and sources of hope: perspectives of family caregivers of people with serious mental illness. Perspect Psychiatr Care 2002; 38(2):61–8.

68. Karp DA, Tanarugsachock V. Mental illness, caregiving, and emotional management. Qual Health Res 2000;10(1):6–25.
69. Tweedell D, Forchuk C, Jewell J, et al. Families' experience during recovery or nonrecovery from psychosis. Arch Psychiatr Nurs 2004;18(1):17–25.
70. Redlich D, Hadas-Lidor N, Weiss P, et al. Mediated learning experience intervention increases hope of family members coping with a relative with severe mental illness. Community Ment Health J 2013;46:409–15.
71. Bandura A. Self-efficacy: the exercise of control. New York: WH Freeman; 1997.
72. Zulkosky K. Self-efficacy: a concept analysis. Nurs Forum 2009;44(2):93–102.
73. Antonovsky A. Health, stress, and coping. San Francisco (CA): Jossey-Bass; 1979.
74. Weimand BM, Hedelin B, Sallstrom C, et al. Burden and health in relatives of persons with severe mental illness: a Norwegian cross-sectional study. Issues Ment Health Nurs 2010;31:804–15.
75. Rosenbaum M. Learned resourcefulness on coping skills, self-control, and adaptive behavior. New York: Springer Publishing Company; 1990.
76. Nadler A. Help-seeking behavior as a coping resource. In: Rosenbaum M, editor. Learned resourcefulness: on coping skills, self-control, and adaptive behavior. New York: Springer; 1990.
77. Zauszniewski JA. Resourcefulness. In: Fitzpatrick JJ, Wallace M, editors. Encyclopedia of nursing research. New York: Spring Publishing Company; 2006.
78. Bekhet A, Johnson N, Zauszniewski JA. Resilience in family members of persons with autism spectrum disorder: a review of the literature. Issues Ment Health Nurs 2012;33(10):650–6.
79. Cherry M, Salmon P, Dickson J, et al. Factors influencing the resilience of carers of individuals with dementia. Rev Clin Gerontol 2013;23(4):251–66.
80. Zauszniewski JA, Bekhet AK, Suresky MJ. Resilience in family members of persons with serious mental illness. Nurs Clin North Am 2010;45(4):613–26.

Special Article: Teaching Clinical Interviewing Skills Using Role-Playing: Conveying Empathy to Performing a Suicide Assessment

Teaching Clinical Interviewing Skills Using Role-Playing: Conveying Empathy to Performing a Suicide Assessment

A Primer for Individual Role-Playing and Scripted Group Role-Playing

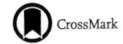

Shawn Christopher Shea, MD[a],*, Christine Barney, MD[b]

KEYWORDS

- Role-playing • Scripted group role-playing • Clinical interviewing
- Suicide assessment • Chronological Assessment of Suicide Events (CASE Approach)

KEY POINTS

- Clinical interviewing skills can be experientially taught and skill retention tested using both traditional individual role-playing and an innovation known as scripted group role-playing (SGRP).
- Recent strategies for enhancing individual role-playing include: improved reverse role-playing; approaches for decreasing trainee anxiety; constructively handling unexpected consequences of role-playing; more realistic patient portrayals.
- SGRP allows supervisors to experientially train up to 28 trainees *simultaneously* in interviewing tasks as complex as sensitively eliciting suicidal ideation and uncovering domestic violence.
- SGRP essentially eliminates "acting" from role-playing resulting in several educational achievements including: striking increase in trainee acceptance and satisfaction with role-playing; markedly more effective use of training time.
- SGRP holds promise for training and nationally certifying psychiatric residents, graduate students, and medical/nursing students in essential interviewing skills such as suicide assessment.

[a] Training Institute for Suicide Assessment and Clinical Interviewing (TISA), 104 Stoney Brook Road, Newbury, NH 03255, USA; [b] 2456 Christian Street, Suite 202, White River Junction, VT 05001, USA
* Corresponding author.
E-mail address: shea@suicideassessment.com; http://www.suicideassessment.com

Psychiatr Clin N Am 38 (2015) 147–183
http://dx.doi.org/10.1016/j.psc.2014.10.001
0193-953X/15/$ – see front matter

Time pressure on busy trainees, who work within capped hours of service, and on busy supervisors, who need to maintain clinical hours to generate their salaries, places a premium on efficiency in training students to master clinical skills. Just as surgical trainees sometimes practice surgical skills in laboratory settings to master basic techniques before performing them on patients,[1] graduate students from all disciplines can benefit from less stressful training situations that focus on specific skill sets through the use of individualized role-playing by skilled coaches. In addition, it now is commonplace for clinical institutions such as community mental health centers, inpatient units, and crisis call centers to provide ongoing training for both new and experienced staff using role-playing to ensure quality assurance.

Role-playing has a major advantage over the use of mere didactics, because it requires a level of understanding that must be translated into actual behavioral practice and subsequent demonstration of the interviewing skills. With the advent of sophisticated applications of role-playing (such as microtraining,[2,3] macrotraining,[4] and scripted group role-playing [SGRP] as introduced in this article), core engagement techniques, in addition to complex interviewing tasks such as transforming crises, eliciting symptoms for accurate diagnosis, and uncovering suicidal ideation, can be taught to a level of competence. Such quality assurance of performance standards is outranked only by direct observation of the student with an actual patient. The freedom from actual clinical demand may reduce the stress level in the learning phase, so that mistakes can be corrected without fear of dire consequences.

Through role-playing, a supervisor can create multiple iterations of the desired skill until competence is obtained. The skill training can subsequently advance in intensity and complexity, including chances to practice using the skill with the supervisor playing the role of resistant clients. Practice continues until the trainer and trainee are confident that the skill is understood and is accessible on demand, and that the trainee is beginning to feel comfortable with its use. Arising from the sound foundation created by role-playing, further skill enhancement can occur if the supervisor has the opportunity to observe the trainee using the techniques with an actual patient, ensuring that the acquired skill has been generalized to clinical practice. Once again, this type of rigorous training has similarities to the sophisticated development of surgeons who achieve proficiency through the intense repetition of skills with patients while being monitored by skilled senior staff.

Using role-playing effectively is not an easy task. If not done well, its results can be disappointing. Moreover, using role-playing is not every instructor's cup of tea; for some teachers it is simply not going to be a good fit. Nevertheless, we believe that many supervisors, even some who initially may feel uncomfortable with it, can be taught to use role-playing successfully and with great enjoyment.

Indeed, we have found role-playing to be one of our most enjoyable of teaching formats. As the developer of macrotraining, I (S.C.S.) have been studying role-playing and serial role-playing intensively for almost 30 years. My coauthor (C.B.) has used role-playing for nearly 20 years as part of the Dartmouth Interviewing Mentorship Program. Together we hope to provide a user-friendly primer that introduces a variety of practical considerations for using role-playing fruitfully in both the individual and group format.

This article focuses on 2 distinct aspects of role-playing: the use of role-playing with individuals and its use with groups of trainees. In Part 1 we address how to perform a single generic role-play well, whether it is used in a simple application, such as offering a student a chance to practice interviewing skills, or in more sophisticated applications, such as microtraining and macrotraining, whereby the goal is to teach interviewing techniques and/or complex interviewing strategies to levels of verifiable competence. Our focus is on practical methods of creating believable role-plays and how to use them to teach specific interviewing skills strategically, while always carefully trying to decrease any anxieties the trainee may have about role-playing itself.

In Part 2, this updated article proffers the opportunity to introduce to the literature an innovative training strategy known as scripted group role-playing (SGRP), a topic not addressed in the original article. SGRP introduces a role-playing format that allows each member of an audience to learn and practice, to an enhanced level of expertise, complex interviewing strategies as might be needed in exploring topics such as suicidal ideation or domestic violence. The second author (C.B.) was not involved in the creation or development of SGRP. Consequently, I (S.C.S.) was the sole author of Part 2, where the benefits, uses, and tips for utilizing SGRP are described in detail.

This informal article is neither a research article nor an academic review: it is a sharing of practical knowledge from teacher to teacher, a hands-on manual of sorts, drawn from our own experience. We do not pretend to have all the answers, and we would love to hear from you of any new ideas you have.

In Part 1, regarding individual role-playing, the approach is 6-fold:

1. To provide a brief history of the varied uses of role-playing
2. To describe the unique training advantages that role-playing offers
3. To delineate some specific tips for role-playing more effectively and for transforming potential problems
4. To address some unexpected consequences of role-playing
5. To provide tips for creating realistic role-playing characters
6. To suggest a list of specific interviewing skills that can be particularly well addressed by role-playing

In Part 2, regarding role-playing used in groups, the approach is 5-fold:

1. To address the significant and complex problems that arise when role-playing is utilized within a group format as opposed to its use with a single trainee
2. To introduce SGRP, which addresses these problems by proffering a style of role-playing that has been well received by trainees for teaching complex interviewing tasks (such as eliciting suicidal ideation) in an effective fashion in a psychologically safe environment
3. To provide a model of how trainers can utilize SGRP to train clinicians to use the Chronological Assessment of Suicide Events (CASE Approach), an innovative interviewing strategy for eliciting suicidal ideation and intent
4. To provide initial empirical data on trainee satisfaction with SGRP
5. To provide practical tips in utilizing SGRP and designing scripted group role plays

PART 1. EFFECTIVE USE OF ROLE-PLAYING WITH A SINGLE TRAINEE
A Brief History of Role-Playing

Role-playing has become a popular and ubiquitous method of training interviewing skills. It is used for training clinicians in numerous disciplines, including medical students, nursing students, psychiatric residents, and residents from other specialties such as primary care and internal medicine, and for training graduate students in techniques of counseling, clinical psychology, social work, and substance abuse counseling. Role-playing also is used as a method of ongoing quality assurance for staff at hospitals, mental health centers, and crisis call centers. Its use can be broken into 3 broad categories.

In its simplest form, clinical instructors use role-playing to provide opportunities for students to practice interviewing skills in an experiential fashion (and in a safe environment where there are no clinical ramifications). In this setting, creative instructors also can use role-playing to present a variety of clients (eg, from diverse socioeconomic and cultural backgrounds and with specific types of psychopathologies or stressors) and differing clinical situations (eg, crisis intervention, ongoing therapy, and inpatient care).

In its more sophisticated and rigorous applications, role-playing can be used to train a single specific interviewing technique, such as using an open-ended question, to a point of behavioral competence (microtraining) or to train complex interviewing strategies, such as eliciting suicidal ideation or uncovering a history of domestic violence, also to a level of behavioral competence (macrotraining).

Another sophisticated use of role-playing is the use of standardized patients (role-played by actors, patients, or instructors) to measure behavioral skills and/or provide feedback about the impact of the student's interviewing style.

The broad utility of role-playing is reflected in the wide range and great number of articles studying or reviewing its use in all three of the categories described, including such remarkably diverse settings as nonmedical classrooms for distance learning in Germany,[5] improving the interest and retention of students exploring careers in mental health research,[6] training primary care residents in interviewing,[7] trouble-shooting the cooperative function of medical teams,[8] addressing patient safety issues and preventive steps by simulating situations that have gone awry,[9] and evaluating sophisticated urologic procedures.[10] A nursing review offers concise cautionary notes regarding the challenges of designing effective simulations,[11] and a Belgian study on teaching communication to medical students provides a candid summary after 6 years of training with a small-group format.[12]

Two advances in role-playing, microtraining and macrotraining, warrant more detailed attention. In the 1960s Ivey[2] developed a sophisticated form of role-playing termed microtraining (also called "microcounseling"), which revolutionized role-playing as an educational tool. Ivey focused on faithfully transmitting one interviewing technique at a time to a student. He realized that providing didactic teaching would not be sufficient to pass on such a behavioral skill, nor would the "loose" practicing of the skill using role-playing. Ivey believed that the trainer must address the skill through the use of modeling and serial role-playing to ensure accurate learning, consolidation of the skill, and generalization of the skill to actual clients, and to enhance the likelihood of long-term retention of the skill at a level of mastery. Ivey's focus was not just on "practice"; it was on practicing until true competence had been shown. His paradigm of microtraining achieved this goal through serial role-playings of a single interviewing technique until it had been consolidated and generalized by the student.

In classic microtraining, the interview question or behavior to be trained must be well defined behaviorally, and usually is described in a manual and modeled on videotape. Some students may be able to "test-out" of the session if they can demonstrate the skill in question. For those who do not know or have not mastered the skill, a microtraining session is used. The trainer focuses on one skill at a time (eg, the use of open-ended questions, empathic statements, or reflecting statements).

After brief reading and a few minutes of didactics enhanced by modeling (often by watching a video), the trainee learns the specific skill through role-playing until the trainer is comfortable that the trainee can demonstrate the skill to a level of competence. In a brief period of time, often 6 to 7 minutes, the trainee practices and consolidates the newly acquired skill using serial role-playing as many times as possible. If time allows, new role-playing incidents with different types of clients are introduced to determine whether the trainee can generalize the newly acquired interviewing skill.

Ivey transformed role-playing from an educational tool that was loosely applied by trainers into an educational technology whereby he delineated specific behaviors by instructors who used role-playing to enhance and consolidate the learning to the point that the trainee could demonstrate actual clinical competence in the pertinent interviewing technique. Ivey did more than speculate: he went in search of empirical data that his training ideas withstood scrutiny. As a result, microcounseling has a large evidence base and may well represent the best-documented interviewing training technique at mentors' disposal. Its evidence base has been accumulating for decades.[13] A review by Daniels[14] found more than 450 studies documenting its efficacy.

My colleagues and I developed the next evolution in role-playing, macrotraining, in the mid-1980s. A practical monograph that describes effective methods for using macrotraining was published in a previous issue of the *Psychiatric Clinics of North America*.[4] Although an interview is composed of individual techniques amenable to microtraining, in the real world of clinical interviewing these techniques do not exist in isolation but always are integrated into specific interviewing tasks. Such tasks often revolve around the gathering of a specific database while maintaining engagement with the client. Typical interviewing tasks (all of which can be taught via macrotraining) might include gathering a picture of symptoms to make a differential diagnosis, eliciting information related to a drug and alcohol history, uncovering information related to interpersonal functioning and social history, and eliciting suicidal ideation. Especially with sensitive topics such as domestic violence, incest, and suicidal ideation, it becomes critical for clinicians to be able to ask questions about difficult-to-share material while simultaneously attending to and nurturing the therapeutic alliance.

Microtraining is effective for teaching individual interviewing techniques, especially those techniques vital to engagement, such as attending behavior and communicating empathy, and using open-ended questions, reflecting statements, and summarizing statements. The next question was whether one could delineate a complex interviewing task such as eliciting suicidal ideation into single small steps that eventually flowed into a larger sequence of effective questioning. If so, could this simplification of the complexities of a real-life interviewing task, such as uncovering incest, be amenable to the serial use of microtraining in each of the steps of the process until the trainee could perform the entire interview flexibly and accurately?

The goal of macrotraining is to teach such complex interviewing strategies to a level of competence in a single session, using serial role-playing of sequences of questions. Complicated interviewing tasks such as eliciting suicidal ideation, planning, and intent often are composed of numerous questions and strategies rather than a single technique as taught in microtraining. Consequently, macrotraining sessions typically last 30 minutes to 4 hours.

Macrotraining was designed both to teach the wording and sequencing of specific types of questions and to allow the trainer, by directly observing the interviewer's tone of voice and use of other nonverbal communications, to ensure that the questions are asked in an engaging fashion.

Thus, while teaching the sequential questioning involved in a complex interviewing strategy, the macrotrainer can ensure that all of the critical basic engagement skills classically taught in microtraining are being used effectively. To date, the most striking use of macrotraining is the teaching of the widely used interviewing strategy for eliciting suicidal ideation, intent, and behaviors known as the **C**hronological **A**ssessment of **S**uicide **E**vents (the CASE Approach).[15] The goal is to make sure that all trainees can demonstrate proficiency in this key clinical task before graduation. Macrotraining has been successfully utilized to certify clinicians in the use of the CASE Approach since the late 1990s.[16]

Before closing our brief history of role-playing, we refer the reader to the third sophisticated use of role-playing: the use of standardized patients for the testing of behavioral skills. Perhaps the best example of this use has been the development of the Objective Structured Clinical Examination, a tool frequently used in medical student and allied health education.[17]

The Benefits of Role-Playing as an Educational Tool

To use role-playing effectively, the first thing a trainer needs is belief—belief that role-playing works and that role-playing provides some specific and unique educational opportunities not available with more traditional methods of teaching. In this section we share a series of benefits to the use of role-playing. Let us begin by sharing one of our favorite techniques, "reverse role-playing," because it nicely illustrates the unique educational power of role-playing. Two definitions are helpful. "Standard role-playing" occurs when the trainer portrays a patient and the student is asked to be the interviewer (practicing the skill in question). "Reverse role-playing" occurs when the trainer and the student reverse roles. In reverse role-playing, the trainer interviews and the student portrays the client. Reverse role-playing is described here in some detail, because it demonstrates what role-playing can accomplish that simply is not possible through didactics, reading material, or even video supervision.

We think you will find that the rotation of roles between the trainer and the student can be beneficial in a variety of situations. In its simplest application, it is used when a trainee is unfamiliar with the relevant skill. Reverse role-playing allows the trainer to model the skill for the trainee at the outset, so the expected target behavior is clear.

Another advantage of reverse role-playing, especially when used early in a session, is that it demonstrates that the trainer is willing "to be put on the spot". In fact, if you do not perform the interviewing technique as well as you wanted, a comment such as, "Boy, I wish I had done that a little differently. Maybe this would have been better. What do you think?" can go a long way toward establishing rapport with the trainee.

We often encourage students to critique our techniques. This openness to feedback conveys a genuine desire for ongoing learning and also models for trainees the importance of asking for feedback when teaching or when conducting therapy itself. In essence, reverse role-playing provides a potent metacommunication of nonhierarchical learning that we believe is communicated most convincingly through reverse role-playing.

There is an even more powerful use of reverse role-playing. Sometimes a trainer encounters a student who does not really believe in the efficacy of an interviewing technique that is being taught. Ultimately, perhaps, the trainer and the student will have to agree to disagree. There is no cookbook way to interview, and we all select interview techniques we enjoy using. On the other hand, the student's hesitancy sometimes is based on inaccurate information or on an erroneous assumption. In such instances, reverse role-playing may provide a valuable tool for transforming the resistance.

Supervisees often are more willing to use new skills once they have felt their impact by playing the patient's role. By being on the receiving end of the technique, they have direct experience with which to reassess their projected fears or misgivings. For example, they might be afraid that the interviewing technique will not work or will be disengaging. If their personal experience in the reverse role-playing is to the contrary, the misgivings dissolve. The following is a more specific example.

As experienced clinicians, we all know that sometimes overly loquacious clients or markedly tangential clients must be redirected and that doing so sometimes requires interrupting the client. Some students are reluctant to use such appropriate interruptions, because they fear that such an intervention is rude and risks disengagement.

This situation is ideal for the use of reverse role-playing whereby the student is asked to portray a wandering client while the trainer uses skilled interruptions effectively to structure the trainee's "client" without causing disengagement. At the end of the reverse role-playing, the student will have learned from direct experience that the structuring by the interviewer felt fine. There can be no more convincing argument than uncovering the truth for oneself.

We often introduce this exercise by saying, "Let's do a role-play in which you play the wandering patient, and I use the structuring techniques; you can see how it actually feels." We also point out to the resident that patients generally want to provide the information that the clinician needs to help them, but patients do not necessarily know what that information is. The structuring helps, and many patients feel more comfortable if the clinician deftly provides cues for when to move to different aspects of a particular topic or even to a brand new topic. The patient actually might feel at sea if the interviewer simply remains nondirective during the main body of the interview.

The following example from the second author's (C.B.) experience shows the striking power of reverse role-playing to transform a learning disagreement by allowing the trainee to experience the interview strategy from the receiving end. One of her psychiatric residents imagined that a victim of domestic violence would find an exploration of some of the details of the violent incident intrusive in an initial interview, especially if there was an effort to delineate the details of the extent of the partner's violence to date. After she used reverse role-playing (during which the trainee assumed the role of the victim) to demonstrate how to uncover such information sensitively, the trainee found it more credible that a person could reasonably tolerate such questioning. The resident even understood, from her own personal feelings during the reverse role-playing, that a patient actually might feel relief that someone finally understood enough to realize how bad things had become. C.B. tacitly demonstrated this knowledge by asking questions that could come only from knowledge of how abuse progresses.

At this point, some fine-tuning information was given to the resident on what type of information needed to be uncovered in such situations and how to do so in a sensitive fashion. Then standard role-playing was used whereby the resident could practice the techniques. Fortuitously, in a follow-up session of supervision in which Barney observed the resident doing a scheduled intake interview, the patient had a significant history of domestic violence. To her credit, the resident managed to sculpt the region well, uncovering pertinent bits of information and doing so in a competent and engaging fashion. After the patient left the interview room she commented on the resident's success, hoping to reinforce it so that it might become part of the resident's ongoing repertoire of skills.

The benefits of role-playing are extensive and fall into the following categories:

1. Assessing the student's skills accurately
2. Building confidence and consolidating skills
3. Broadening case material
4. Learning to transform angry and awkward moments
5. Strengthening clinical reasoning
6. Modeling new interviewing techniques

7. Gaining comfort with new interviewing skills
8. Enhancing videotape supervision

Assessing skills accurately

One of the most important advantages of role-playing is the direct observation of a student's skills to assure that competence is present. No student can be fully aware of what he or she is doing while doing it; therefore, a student's report that a technique is being done well may or may not be accurate. Indeed, a student may be saying the correct words but may accompany the technique with nonverbal behaviors that are disengaging or have a poor sense of timing. In another spectrum, cognitive knowledge base, role-playing can help establish the limits of the supervisee's knowledge and experience. To explore a given region of data, such as the *Diagnostic and Statistical Manual of Mental Disorders*, 5th edition (DSM-5) criteria of a specific diagnosis or the information required in a sound social history, the trainee must be familiar with the body of information to be elicited and must be able to consider which questions to ask to gather that data most efficiently. Role-playing uncovers any weaknesses in this knowledge base quickly and clearly.

Paradoxically, in a few instances role-playing can give a more accurate representation of skill competency than a video of a student's interview with an actual patient, a point seldom addressed in the literature. Videos can create artifacts that may result from the trainee's anxiety about being filmed, with a resulting loss of spontaneity or natural employment of interpersonal skills, a problem we refer to as "video freeze." In other instances, specific singular issues that may have been prompted by the particular patient in the video may detract from the student's overall display of skill. For instance, a clinician who normally is adept at gathering information regarding diagnosis in a sensitive fashion may appear stilted if this particular patient was hostile early in the interview, during the filming, and had thrown the student off balance. This situation on the video will of course focus the trainer's attention immediately on helping the student deal with hostility, but it also may give an inaccurate portrayal of the student's typical diagnostic skills. It may help to role-play the part of a nonhostile interview in which the student's diagnostic skills would be needed, to determine whether the skill is truly lacking or was merely compromised by the presence of the camera.

Videos also may lead to inaccurate overestimation of a trainee's knowledge base; for example, if a frequently hospitalized patient was taped and spontaneously gave information so readily that little skill was required by the interviewer, the interviewer might appear artificially talented at obtaining a robust database.

Building confidence and consolidating skills

One of the most powerful advantages of role-playing is the consolidation of skill through repetition. Repetition (with slight variation to avoid boredom) is the cornerstone of both the microtraining of single skills and the macrotraining of complex interviewing sequences. Such consolidation can play a pivotal role in enhancing the likelihood that the student will generalize the interviewing skill and maintain it over time.

Similarly, it may be worthwhile to role-play some of the trainee's strengths and reinforce them. Such role-playing of "safe skills" may convince a student who is wary of role-playing that it is a reasonably comfortable experience with minimal attached stress. Practicing strengths also can protect against the specific supervisory misstep of focusing too much on the acquisition of new skills while a recently acquired skill fades through lack of positive reenforcement from the trainer.

Broadening case material

No matter what the inherent quality of the program in which a student is trained, there will be some sampling bias among the patient types the student encounters. For instance, programs may vary in how often the student works with people suffering from acute psychotic episodes, war-related posttraumatic stress disorder, or eating disorders or encounters with clients from minority cultures. Role-playing of different situations with which students are less familiar or unacquainted will help them feel more prepared when they encounter a novel patient complaint or type of presentation. Although attempting to prepare a student for all rarely encountered situations is impractical, there is utility in screening the trainee's experience to find out if there are common clinical problems that the trainee is underprepared to handle effectively.

Learning to transform angry and awkward moments

Even a supervisor who is sitting in on interviews, watching through a one-way mirror, or routinely reviewing video sessions may never see the student handling certain difficult situations. Two key difficult situations are angry exchanges and awkward questions from clients directed to the interviewer, such as, "Do you believe it is ever okay to kill yourself?" or "Do you believe in God?" or "What is your sexual orientation?" or "Do you believe me?" (asked by a patient regarding his or her own delusional belief).

Learning to handle anger gracefully and nondefensively or to respond appropriately to awkward questions highlights two other uses of role-playing. Role-playing may well be the most effective method for training the student in this particular set of clinical skills. Role-playing allows the student to address a specific awkward moment repeatedly while experimenting with different types of responses in a totally safe environment. It gives ample time for the student to share personal feelings generated by the awkward moment that may need to be discussed before effective training can continue. Once the student becomes comfortable with various ways of handling the awkward moment, the skill can be consolidated through an iteration of targeted role-plays.

Strengthening clinical reasoning

As the alliance of the supervisor/supervisee pair develops over time, the trainer can present the trainee with increasing levels of challenge in their role-playing. This graduated challenge offers the trainer a better chance to assess and improve the student's ability to evaluate clinical situations more astutely, and to solve problems more effectively in various hypothetical situations.

Role-plays can provide a forum for inquiry and gaining mastery, and motivated trainees often bring clinical material from their on-call or clinic experiences to interviewing supervision. In such instances, the trainer can discuss the trainee's concerns and then collaborate to develop strategies for the trainee to try out, subsequently using role-playing created on the spot to match the trainee's concerns. Reverse role-playing can offer the trainee a chance to see exactly what the proposed interviewing technique feels like.

Supervisors can draw from their own experience to provide training in related but less commonly encountered issues, so that trainees can be better prepared to handle the unexpected. With increasing comfort in the technique, trainees can minimize the time spent discussing, "What should I do if…?" Instead, they are more eager to jump into role-playing to see what the suggested intervention might offer.

Modeling new interviewing techniques

"A picture is worth a thousand words" is eminently applicable to learning interviewing and psychotherapy skills. As mentioned earlier, reverse role-playing is invaluable in this regard when videotaped illustrations of technique are not available. Reverse role-playing also has the advantage of immediately modeling a technique with the exact type of client with whom the trainee encountered difficulties, a technique not available from a premade video.

Gaining comfort with new interviewing skills

Many of the factors that make role-playing ideal for teaching new interviewing skills have been touched on in the discussion of the uses of role-playing. An advantage that has not yet been noted is that the ability to practice a focused technique in multiple iterations can reduce the trainee's experience of "stage fright" or "the mind going blank" when trying something new, and can push the trainee to address specific fears or weaknesses. Role-playing provides a safe arena in which the student realizes that techniques are being practiced and that errors are expected and acceptable, and in which the training dyad can address issues requested by the student and at the student's own pace. To use role-playing to teach complex new interviewing skills and strategies to a level of competence, we once again direct you to the educational technologies of microtraining[2] and macrotraining.[4]

Enhancing video supervision

Video supervision can be enhanced if supervisor is skilled in the use of role-playing, microtraining, and macrotraining. We call such supervision "role-play–enhanced video supervision." If a particular problem for which a specific interviewing technique could be useful is spotted during video supervision, it can be highly effective to replay the relevant segment, describe the skill, and immediately follow the demonstration with role-playing to try out the new technique. Subsequent role-playing can be used to consolidate the learning.

When facilic supervision (a supervision language and schematic shorthand for spotting problems with how residents structure interviews and helping them to create conversationally graceful transitions between topics)[18,19] is used in conjunction with filming video, new avenues for the productive use of role-playing arise. If the trainer sees on the video that the resident has problems gracefully exploring a specific diagnostic region, this problem can be highlighted, and the trainer, using reverse role-playing, can immediately model more effective ways for naturalistically exploring the desired symptoms. The trainee then can try out the new techniques in standard role-playing.

At times, a student's skill deficit may be related to emotionally charged material or countertransferential feelings (eg, a student routinely does a poor exploration of the region of substance abuse related to the student's father suffering from alcoholism). In such cases, the use of interpersonal process recall[20] can help the trainee better address the indicated clinical skills. This triadic combination of video, interpersonal process recall, and role-playing can be powerful.

Some Tips for More Effective Role-Playing

Minimizing anxiety related to role-playing

Students vary significantly in their attitudes toward role-playing, ranging from obvious enthusiasm to intense dislike. The direct observation of one's skills can generate an intense awareness of scrutiny, with a heightened sense of a trainee's vulnerability. We have found a variety of attitudes and methods that can significantly enhance a trainee's sense of appreciation for, and comfort with, role-playing.

With regard to the trainer's attitude, two key attributes have helped guide our actions over the years: humility and fallibility. We manifest these attributes by emphasizing that we are teaching a wide variety of tools to broaden a clinician's options, rather than teaching "the right way" to conduct interviews. We emphasize that we are trying to generate enthusiasm about the power and nuances of clinical interviewing whereby we eagerly invite discussion, differences of opinion, and creative approaches to strategizing. We hope that we are providing the trainee with the tools to engage in a lifelong study and refinement of interviewing process. To re-enforce further that we, too, are learning, and that we, too, make mistakes, we occasionally find it useful to recount our own errors or misfires when a technique that seemed to be indicated did not work well with an individual patient.

Flexibility—knowing what else to try when a given approach is unsuccessful—is a much more useful goal than a robotic repetition of technique. Helping interviewers allow for blunders or gaffes, and even modeling how to apologize to a patient who finds a particular phrase or intervention offensive or disquieting, can help trainees abandon constricting ideas that reduce their humanity, and can allow the appropriate use of their personalities in interviews.

If a student believes that patients are fragile and apt to fall apart unless the interviewer displays perfect empathy, he or she may be reluctant to offer any empathic statements for fear of being out of synch with the patient. Casting off the myths that the trainer is a perfect interviewer, or that perfection is even an achievable goal in the real world of clinical interviewing, can reduce the burdens under which particularly anxious or high-achieving trainees may labor.

Before beginning role-playing, we recommend asking, "Have you ever done role-playing, and what was it like for you?" Many students have had good experiences, but a sizable number have not, especially if they have experienced poorly executed role-playing. Typical biases include the idea that role-playing is silly, unrealistic, artificial, useless, or makes one feel uncomfortable[4]. That is quite a list! It is better to have these concerns on the table than constantly undermining the role-playing experience as one proceeds. Once doubts are out on the table, the supervisor has the opportunity to transform such biases or to reduce them. When an occasional trainee expresses strong misgivings about role-playing, we recommend beginning by acknowledging and accepting his or her concerns with a comment such as:

> You know, you are absolutely right. Role-playing can really be pretty much a waste of time. I personally had some bad experiences with it in my training, where it just didn't do anything for me. What I've learned over the years is that there are good ways to do it and not so good ways, and I think I've learned a lot of ways to make it work well. Part of the trick is making the patients seem real, and I've gotten pretty good at that. You'll have to let me know if I'm not believable in a given role, but I've got some pretty interesting patients to show you that are based directly on my own clinical practice.

We also find it useful to describe gently (using soft sell, not hard sell) some of the unique advantages to role-playing to the trainee:

1. Role-playing allows the role-players to study a specific type of clinical situation that may occur only sporadically with actual patients (eg, a patient describing delusions), whenever they wish, and as often as they wish.
2. Role-players can go at their own pace, and the trainee will determine what pace is best.
3. Role-players can practice whatever they want.
4. Role-players have the luxury of focusing on only one clinical interviewing technique at a time.

5. There are absolutely no clinical pressures on role-players because they are merely practicing. There is no real patient in the room, and any mistakes either role-player makes have no ramifications.

After the very first role-play during a training session, we also recommend asking, "How did that go for you?" Depending on the student's answer, we might ask, "Is there anything we might do to make this even more comfortable or useful for you?"

In the experience of the second author's (C.B.) work with trainees and with clients, she feels indebted to the work of the behavioral psychologist Pryor.[20] Pryor's work in positive reinforcement training across multiple species is instructive in basic principles for creating a safe, effective, and enjoyable environment for behavioral change. She has convincing experience that establishes the need for:

1. Having clear expectations
2. Marking the desired behavior precisely as it emerges
3. Recognizing initial steps that are approximations toward the desired goal
4. Gradually raising the bar on the skill level of the performance that is needed to get recognition
5. Eliminating expression of the trainer's frustration to the subject
6. Rewarding correct behavior
7. Attending to the subject's fatigue or frustration, and ending the training session on a positive note with a skill that is under mastery

Pryor also offers an intriguing approach toward reducing performance anxiety. She notes that training the last step in a behavioral sequence first can be a key to successful completion of a behavioral chain, especially when learning this last skill set to competence assures recognition and reward.

The principle in such training "backward from the end" is that the most rehearsed skill set (because the trainee has role-played it to competence) and, therefore, the area of greatest confidence becomes something that the trainee is moving toward during the remainder of the role-playing sessions. Rather than experiencing anticipatory anxiety, the trainee anticipates the relief of approaching a comfort zone.

(Clinicians who use positive imagery and hypnosis may see a parallel to the technique for decreasing anticipatory anxiety or phobic avoidance whereby clients imagine safety from a feared task by rehearsing a successful conclusion and then develop the sequence in reverse. For example, a patient who has airplane phobia could begin by picturing a successful landing and getting off the plane and then work backward in small steps, eventually picturing the sequence from the beginning, at the stage of preparing to leave for the airport.)

Back to interview training, suppose you were training a resident to do an entire initial interview, and he or she has a history of trouble helping patients to close down at the end of an interview. You might start by role-playing the closing of the interview first, with the trainee practicing the closing until competence is achieved while you provide positive feedback with each element of improvement to instill more confidence. From this point onward, as you begin training the resident, in steps, for the rest of the interview, the trainee always will know that he or she is moving toward a task (the closing of the interview) with which the student now feels comfortable and competent. This technique might be helpful for students with performance anxiety about finishing on time, gathering enough data, or being able to bring the interview to an acceptable close.

Another aspect of decreasing anxiety deals with addressing the emotional impact of the role-playing as the session goes on. For instance, it is sometimes best to end role-playing early if the trainee seems to be exhausted or disheartened by not "getting it right." Ideally the trainer can go back to an earlier role-playing scenario that the trainee fulfilled well, ensuring that the supervision session ends on a note of success. At other times, one may shift completely away from role-playing and use didactics, in addition to a sense of humor, to bring the session to a nonthreatening and comfortable end.

Another aspect of reducing anxiety relates not to the session at hand but to the use of ongoing role-playing with a student whom one may be supervising over a longer period, as when a trainer/trainee pair is sustained over the course of a year. Here a new principle enters the picture. Within the safety of a well-developed longitudinal relationship with the supervisor, a trainee may be able to tolerate and derive benefit from deeper scrutiny.

In short-term role-playing training, one usually focuses on the exact wording and sequencing of behaviorally specific interview techniques and strategies. Attitudes conveyed by the interviewer, however, can have a great impact on how well that interviewer is received by a given patient. These attitudes are transmitted through qualities such as tone of voice, timing of intervention, other nonverbal mannerisms, and the basic attributes of the resident's personality. (Some residents can come across as self-important "big shots" or as poor listeners who seem as though they do not "really care"; others may be prone to making narcissistic insults or have a paternalistic demeanor.) Clearly it is important to address these problems. We have found that the tone of the delivery of our feedback and our ability to maintain a respectful attitude are important in helping residents with such delicate matters that reflect back on their personality structures.

Equally important, during longitudinal supervision, we purposefully avoid focusing on many such nonverbal communication problems until much later in the year, to allow more time for rapport to be established before trying to alter behaviors that the trainee might view as too personal or potentially invasive. Once a safe supervisory relationship has become well established over months, it sometimes is surprising how many of these more delicate matters can be addressed successfully through direct discussion and also through role-playing.

You may encounter a few trainees who have remarkably elevated anxiety related to role-playing. In a rare instance, a trainee may have a true social phobia with an intense fear of "performing" any task whereby he or she will be observed directly. If you encounter such a situation, role-playing may be counterproductive, and the teaching of the interview strategy that was the subject of the role-playing session may be approached better in less directly observed ways while helping the trainee seek professional help for the ongoing social phobia.

Effectively interrupting the role-playing to make a teaching point

In theory, one can wait to provide feedback to the trainee until the role-playing is completed, and there are good reasons for doing so in specific settings. On the other hand, it is much more common to want to provide immediate feedback, especially if the trainee is doing a technique poorly. One reason for such prompt interruption is that one does not want the trainee to consolidate the error by repetition. Also, from a behavioral learning perspective, it can be more advantageous to provide corrective feedback as soon as possible after the problematic behavior and to reward good behavior promptly. We refer to this interruption of role-playing as "marking" the role-play.

In behavior modification with nonhuman animals, a clicker device often is used to mark a behavior as soon as it happens.[21] Although such a device could be used as a marker in role-playing, we have found it much easier to agree on a specific hand signal, which either the trainer or the trainee can use at any time, to stop the role-playing. Such a hand signal functions like a time-out signal used to call for a break in the action of a football game.

Unless a time-out has been called, the dyad remains in role at all times. Students who are hesitant to do role-playing are notorious for breaking out of role often, greatly diminishing the likelihood that a realistic feeling will begin to unfold. This problem can be addressed easily by enforcing the norm that, unless a time-out is called, both parties will remain in role. It cannot be overemphasized that, for role-playing to become "real" to the participants, it is critical that they stay in role unless the role-playing has been marked by one of the participants. Trainees benefit greatly when the simulation achieves the emotional intensity that would be generated in an actual clinical interview (eg, the fear of someone with paranoia, the despair of a depressed patient, or the hostile irritability of someone who is manic). If trainees have encountered and mastered such emotionally charged situations during role-playing practice, they are less apt to be disconcerted by them when subsequently encountered in clinical practice.

Even if the student has done a good job, you should try not to smile or nod encouragement, because this action breaks the role-playing: the patient you are portraying would not make such a gesture. You can give simple, on-the-spot positive feedback effectively by marking the session, breaking out of role briefly, and saying something like, "That was a great use of open-ended questions; keep going, and let's see what else you uncover," then returning immediately into role. Such a consistent adherence to the rules of role-playing keeps the sessions on track and realistic, much as sticking to group norms in group therapy is vital to the functioning of the group.

Handling Unexpected Consequences of Role-Playing

Role-playing, by its very nature, is ad lib. A trainer never knows exactly which direction a specific role-play may take, because this direction depends on the student's responses. Spontaneity is the name of the game, sometimes for the good and sometimes for the bad.

On the bad side, the focus of the learning may move unexpectedly to a new topic. Thinking on the fly, with one's plan being to focus on a single teaching point, we as trainers may believe we are training only the topic of focus; however, the trainee is responding to our dialogue and nonverbal behaviors and to the trainee's own internal associations. Although we believe we are training one specific point or technique, and even if we clearly state that intention to the trainee, the student may be detecting something else in the role-playing that is notable for the trainee but may have been unintentional or incidental in the mind of the supervisor. I sometimes ask for questions or comments at the end of a role-playing to see if unintended points were made or if some ambiguity arose.

Unscheduled shifts into new teaching areas are not always problematic. Indeed, as the level of comfort and familiarity between trainee and trainer increases over multiple meetings in a longitudinal supervision, it may become both easy and advantageous to flow with the new direction the trainee takes, addressing serendipitous teaching points that may be very useful to the trainee. One always can return subsequently to the intended teaching point.

Another unintended consequence of role-playing is related to the emotional intensity generated by the role-playing itself. Although many students begin by saying that role-playing does not feel real to them, the situation can become all too real in the hands of a gifted role-player. The evolution of a role suddenly can become compellingly intense, and trainees may use it to put forth some profound or distressing interaction they have had with patients in the past. At other times, the trainer's portrayal of a patient may elicit a reaction in the student that seems excessive, and even a brief inquiry from the trainer may result in the student's revealing an important incident such as incest in the trainee's own life.

Supervisors vary in how they attend to such revelations, by briefly exploring the incident as it relates to its immediate impact on the trainee as a clinician or by referring the trainee to a psychotherapy supervisor whose role more frequently includes dealing with countertransference. Of course, in conjunction with the residency director, a decision sometimes is made to suggest individual therapy if there clearly is a significant area of concern for the trainee's mental health or if the trainee's emotional distress hinders his or her clinical work.

On a much lighter note, however, the most common serendipitous consequence of role-playing is laughter and the use of humor by both the trainer and the trainee. When a role-played patient with manic disinhibition is baiting a young trainee by picking on his or her lack of training or flies into a hysterically funny set of loose associations, sometimes you just have to laugh. If one is at a critical point in teaching a technique, and there is just a bit of a chuckle from the trainee, it often is best simply to stay in character, and the trainee will follow suit. If both parties are struck by a particular spontaneously funny circumstance, it usually is best to mark the session, pull out of role, and laugh with abandon. Such moments can be valuable in creating a comfortable and enjoyable alliance with the student. The humanness of both parties is reassuring and delightfully refreshing.

Tips for Creating Realistic Characters in Role-Playing

The following tips are adapted from the *Training Manual for Macrotrainers*.[22] In role-playing, it often is useful to picture a specific client you have encountered in your practice and to borrow heavily from that client's presentation in your role-playing. In visualizing the client, you should pay particular attention to your memories of the client's hand gestures, tone of voice, rate of speech, and posture. These details often give a stamp of reality to role-playing, because they may be quite different from your own nonverbal mannerisms.

For instance, a patient who has a severe depression generally speaks at a much slower rate than the typical trainer, and this difference should be apparent to the trainee (but will undoubtedly require your conscious effort while in the role).

As you begin to use role-playing regularly, it is useful to prepare a stock set of role-plays from which you can borrow freely. For instance, you may develop readily reproducible characters that portray excessively wandering clients, shut-down clients, the classic client who responds with "I don't know" to every question, a suicidal client with minimal intent and actions, a suicidal client with intense intent and actions taken on his or her suicidal plan, a delusional client, or a client with marked loosening of associations. As you use these personalities over the years, your portrayals can become more vivid and more realistic.

As stated earlier, to help enhance the realism of the role-playing, both parties should stay strictly in role. Always make it plain whether you are in role or out of role, using a hand signal for time-outs as markers. Before you start role-playing, you should take a moment to visualize the role and get into character, then picture what you are going to do, recalling the character or patient who embodies the target quality or history. Proceed with, "Okay let's go," and begin the role-playing. Be sure to think about making your attire congruent with that of the patient being portrayed: you may want to remove items such as ties, scarves, or suit coats.

Usually a couple of minutes are needed for the realism of the role-playing to take hold. Consequently, you should not enter the skill you wish to teach until the role-playing has continued long enough to give the student a feel for the patient you are portraying. Likewise, when first learning how to use role-playing to enhance interviewing skills (and students' role-playing skills do improve), students sometimes fall out of role, falter, or giggle in the early moments of the role-playing. Stay in role! The student will follow suit, greatly speeding up your ability to use role-playing as an effective educational tool.

In teaching more complex interviewing skills, as occurs during macrotraining, you often will create new roles designed specifically to meet the training needs of the student at that exact moment. Once again, it is helpful to try to picture a patient you encountered in the past. A newly minted role may not be as realistic as those you use regularly. That is fine and to be expected. It always is more important to build role-playing that allows the trainee to learn the desired skill than to create an "Oscar-winning" performance.

If you are creating role-playing in which the trainee is to consolidate a skill by practicing the exact skill again, but with a different patient, one should try to make the new patient have a distinctly different personality. We find that recalling the memory of a real patient and focusing on showing distinctive mannerisms (nervously picking at one's nails, twirling hair, or looking down at the floor to avoid eye contact) that differ from the previously portrayed patient makes it much easier to separate adjacent role-playings.

Finally, while you are designing role-playings on the spot, you must keep in mind the guiding principle, "keep it simple." Trainers should aim to teach one skill at a time; be sure you know what the skill you want this particular role-playing to develop in the student and make sure the student is ready to learn that skill. In essence, ensure that you are not asking too much of a particular student: he or she must be ready to move on to the next step. Before you begin role-playing, it is useful to restate the task and ask, "Do you have any questions about what you are trying to do in this role-play?"

Specific Interviewing Skills Well Addressed by Role-Playing

The number of clinical skills well addressed by role-playing is extensive, from interviewing techniques to psychotherapeutic skills, limited only by the behavioral specificity of the techniques and the imaginations of the trainers. Over the years we have found some interviewing techniques and strategies that can be addressed with particular success using role-playings, which are listed here. We feel certain that you will create many more.

1. Individual interviewing techniques (optimally taught through microtraining)
   a. Open-ended questions
   b. Closed-ended questions
   c. Empathic statements
   d. Reflecting statements
   e. Summarizing statements
   f. Gentle commands, qualitative questions, statements of inquiry[19]
   g. Validity techniques
      Behavioral incident[23]
      Gentle assumption[24]
      Shame attenuation, symptom amplification, denial of the specific[22]
   h. Facilitative nonverbal communications (eg, head nodding, forward leaning)

2. Interviewing sequences and strategies (optimally taught through macrotraining)
    a. Sequential use of basic engagement techniques to strengthen the alliance
    b. Scouting training: performing the first 7 minutes of the interview in an engaging fashion with different types of patients, then asking the interviewer to provide his or her plans for shaping the rest of the interview[16]
    c. Effectively handling the flow of questioning while sculpting out a specific DSM-5 diagnosis in a sensitive and comprehensive fashion
    d. Focusing wandering or hypomanic patients
    e. Opening up shut-down or frightened patients
    f. Interviewing psychotic and paranoid patients
    g. Transforming angry moments (including verbally abusive patients)
    h. Nondefensively handling awkward or intrusive questions directed at the clinician
    i. Sensitively and comprehensively eliciting potentially taboo histories:
        Sexual history and sexual orientation
        Domestic violence
        Incest
        Alcohol and substance abuse
        Antisocial, criminal, and homicidal thoughts or behaviors
    j. Eliciting suicidal ideation, planning, intent, and behaviors using the Chronological Assessment of Suicide Events[2,4,15]
    k. Providing psychoeducation
    l. Talking effectively with patients about their medications and addressing their concerns about side effects[25]

PART 2. SCRIPTED GROUP ROLE-PLAYING
Introduction

When role-playing is used in groups, it can be utilized in one of two formats: (1) as a platform for group discussion and/or (2) in a skills enhancement format whereby participants experientially practice interviewing techniques and strategies. When used primarily as a platform for discussion, role-plays (which often involve the instructor as one of the participants) are frequently performed in front of the group as a means of generating discussion and brainstorming. I have used this format repeatedly, and it can be quite powerful. I have used it effectively in groups as large as 120 participants, although it generally works best in significantly smaller groups.

If a trainee is assuming the role of the interviewer in front of a group of other participants, social and performance anxiety can be fairly intense. Indeed, "volunteers" seem to decrease in number as the size of the class increases. It becomes critical to minimize anxiety immediately, with both the class and the volunteers from the class. Although an entire paper could be written addressing the art of running such classes, such a discussion is beyond the scope of this article. However, I would like to share a specific phrasing that I have found to be useful in minimizing performance anxiety in this setting. As the very first volunteer is stepping up to participate in the initial role-play, I often make a comment such as:

I just want to emphasize the purpose of our role-plays today. We are not here to critique John's interview or pass on constructive criticism to John or anyone who helps us out with our role-plays today. Instead we are using the role-plays as a platform to launch our discussions. The role-play will allow us to actually see something that we can tangibly play with. Our goal will be to brainstorm on different ways of handling the situations presented by the clients. Indeed, John may even try out some of our ideas and we will see their pros and cons as they unfold. We will function with the help of John, and all of you who help us out today, as a team that gains a more nuanced understanding of how clients are presenting and the numerous ways in which we can effectively approach specific tasks and challenges. Our role-plays today will provide us with a real-time training field where we can try out our ideas together in a way that is simply not possible in the clinic itself. I think you will find that these role-plays will give us a rich launching pad for discussion and brainstorming. Before we start let's give John a big hand for being the first to help us out and then let's get to work.

Let us now move to the focus of this part of the article, for I want to address the much more challenging and, arguably, more important second format of group role-playing: the skills enhancement format. To make this format useful the trainer must come up with a viable answer to the following question: "Can role-playing be used in a group format to provide immediate constructive feedback that results in skill enhancement to all members of the class?" Three more specific questions frame the challenge more operationally:

1. Can a group format be conducive to providing feedback in a fashion that is enjoyable and minimizes social performance anxiety?
2. Can a productive number of new techniques be taught to all participants in the time available?
3. In addition to single, simple interviewing techniques, can complex interview strategies (such as uncovering suicidal ideation and intent, differential diagnosis, sensitively uncovering incest and other forms of domestic violence) be taught to demonstrable competence in a group format?

Truth be told, not everyone feels that the answer to these questions is "yes."

A sizable chunk of motivated trainees simply do not like role-playing in groups. The roots of their dislike are many and diverse, such as: (1) feeling uncomfortable and "being put on the spot" when asked to be the interviewer in front of colleagues; (2) and acting (as required when role-playing the patient) not being a comfortable skill set for the participant, or; (3) as many participants comment, the "whole thing just feels stupid to me and unrealistic." Indeed there are trainees, as well as subsequent experienced clinicians, who will not attend a workshop if they know beforehand that role-playing is going to be used.

It is important as teachers to accept a primary educational truth: trainees do not learn well if they do not like the training approach with which they are being taught. Period. However, this is not the trainee's fault but the trainer's fault. The trainer of any specific clinical interviewing skill set must determine the fashion in which the trainee is best suited to learn. A significant number of graduate students and professionals find role-playing in a group format to be artificial and an inappropriate medium for their development.

Herein lies the problem and the paradox. Interviewing techniques (such as open-ended questions, empathic statements, and reflecting statements) are core skill sets to master for any graduate from psychiatric residencies and nurse clinician programs to clinical psychology, social work, and counseling graduate programs. In addition, even more strikingly, complex interviewing skills such as eliciting suicidal ideation/intent, uncovering incest/domestic violence, and transforming anger from a patient are critical skills that are needed on a daily basis and may have life-saving implications. Any trainee from such programs should be able to demonstrate proficiency in such complex interviewing skills on graduation, but these skills are often most easily taught and tested via role-playing.

*Micro*training can be used to teach single interviewing skills to competence (Ivey)[2], and *macro*training (Shea)[4] can be used to teach complex interviewing strategies to competence. But the limitation of these *individualized* role-playing approaches is a practical one of immense importance in graduate and postgraduate training: time, not enough of it. Especially with regard to complex and critical interviewing skills such as eliciting suicidal ideation, there may not be enough interested instructors to effectively train to competence each trainee in a specific year of a graduate class in these skills. Such complex skills can be effectively taught with macrotraining but may require several hours to do so per trainee.

Even outside the discipline of mental health, these complex interviewing skills are of immense importance. Who could argue with the idea that all medical, nursing, physician assistant, and clinical pharmacy students should be trained to effectively and sensitively uncover suicidal ideation, when it has been shown repeatedly that more than 50% of all people who die by suicide have seen a physician/primary care provider within 1 month of death[26]? Each of these students could be successfully taught this skill through the use of macrotraining, but macrotraining the elicitation of suicidal ideation and intent can take between 2 and 4 hours per student per instructor.[4] If a specific medical school class consists of 150 students, it is simply not feasible for that school to provide 300 to 600 hours of individualized role-playing despite the fact that suicide assessment is a critical skill set. If this skill set is not learned, the student may be unable to spot serious suicidal intent in his or her subsequent practice with potentially dire results.

The answer must lie in creating a style of role-playing designed specifically for larger groups of trainees who in some fashion "pair off" into smaller role-playing groups (pods) to practice together. As promising as this answer sounds, I would bet that just about any instructor who has ever taught such a class has no doubt encountered the plethora of new obstacles that arise with their use.

First, and foremost, unlike one-on-one role-playing performed alone in the safety of a supervisor's office, performance anxiety can skyrocket in such groups. Trainees can experience anxiety around two entirely different tasks: (1) anxiety related to the performance of the requested interviewing technique or strategy in front of peers, and/or (2) anxiety related to acting the role of a client. Often triggered by these anxieties, a significant number of the trainees will enter the session "dreading role-playing." Unfortunately, especially if the trainee's defense mechanism for handling such anxiety is a passive-aggressive one or is based on a feigned showing of disinterest, problems can quickly metastasize to the entire small learning pod. Just one such trainee in a pod of two or four participants can significantly undercut the learning experience for all participants in the pod. Two such disinterested trainees are basically a death-knell to effective learning for the other participants.

Disinterested trainees are not the only problem. Sometimes, participants who "just *love* role-playing" love role-playing because it gives them a chance to win an Oscar. It has been my experience that such budding actors/actresses seldom pass up on this "chance of a lifetime." These role-players are crying (sometimes real tears), pounding their fists in pain, or creating antagonistic clients who thwart the interviewer at every corner of the role-play.

Because class participant role-players do not know, nor have been trained to know, the exact best fashion in which to play the patient so as to optimize the learning of the colleague practicing the interviewing skill or strategy, the role-playing exercises can become grossly inefficient. Unlike individual skill-enhancement role-playing strategies such as Ivey's microtraining or Shea's macrotraining, whereby the role-playing is being done by the trainer, the role-play's effectiveness is at the whim of the trainee role-player.

The role-plays can quickly become far too long and/or too difficult to do effectively because the role-player has created a client whose psychopathology or communication style would warrant a different interviewing technique than is being practiced.

In contrast to individualized role-playing, arguably the greatest problem in a group format is a markedly, sometimes drastically, reduced amount of time in which the trainer can directly observe each of the participants to provide constructive feedback, as the instructor must be hopping from group to group while all the different groups are practicing simultaneously. If the goal of the training is the passing on of the skills needed to perform a complex interviewing task such as suicide assessment or the uncovering of incest, this problem is formidable.

In the remainder of this article, an innovative style of group role-playing, SGRP, is described as it has been utilized to train clinicians in a widely applied method for uncovering suicidal ideation, planning, actions, and intent: the Chronological Assessment of Suicide Events (the CASE Approach). SGRP has been evolving for nearly 15 years and is now well field tested (some of the results from which are briefly shared herein). Indeed, since 2012 experiential training on the CASE Approach using SGRP[16] has been placed on the Best Practices Registry regarding trainings available on suicide assessment and prevention. The Best Practices Registry was created and is maintained by the Suicide Prevention and Resources Center (SPRC), supported by an ongoing grant from the Substance Abuse and Mental Health Services Administration (SAMHSA).

SGRP offers a new approach to group role-playing that effectively addresses all of the concerns listed earlier. It also answers the "challenging questions" raised earlier in this section with a "yes." In short, SGRP allows a sizable number of participants (up to 28 per class) to be trained to enhanced fidelity in complex interviewing strategies (in this case the elicitation of suicidal ideation, planning, behaviors, and intent) using role-playing in a fashion that is enjoyable to all participants with the exception of a rare few.

My goal is to introduce the reader to the principles of SGRP and foster both an interest in and the tools necessary to begin your own exploration of the use of SGRP in whatever aspect of interviewing you are training, from simple, core interviewing techniques to complex interviewing strategies of your choice. It is not meant to be a manual for the use of SGRP, but I hope it can provide enough information for the reader to make his or her own excursions and experimentations in its use. To achieve this goal I will do the following: (1) review the challenge of training toward fidelity one of the most critical of all interviewing strategies—the elicitation of suicidal ideation; (2) examine the field testing results when SGRP has been applied to this educational task; and (3) describe the core characteristics and principles of SGRP.

Illustration of Scripted Group Role-Playing: Putting Scripted Group Role-Playing to the Test

Using scripted group role-playing to train clinicians in suicide assessment

I will focus here on the use of SGRP in training clinicians to uncover suicidal ideation, planning, behavior, and intent, for four reasons: (1) suicide assessment is one of the most important and daunting of interviewing challenges; (2) a widely acclaimed interviewing strategy, the CASE Approach, has been well delineated in the literature; (3) the CASE Approach is a sophisticated interview strategy requiring the use of seven different interviewing techniques woven into a variety of different interviewing strategies—this degree of sophistication highlights the ability of SGRP to train a large number of clinicians to a level of enhanced skill in a complex interviewing strategy; and (4)

SGRP has been utilized and field tested extensively in the training of clinicians across disciplines and experience groups with regard to the CASE Approach.

The CASE Approach was first described in the literature in 1998 by its innovator Shea[19,27] and has subsequently been received enthusiastically among mental health professionals, substance abuse counselors, college and high school counselors, primary care clinicians, the military and Veterans Affairs (VA) systems, and the correctional profession.[15,28-38] The CASE Approach is presented routinely as a core clinical course at the annual meetings of the American Association of Suicidology[39] and is recommended as a resource for telephone crisis providers by the National Suicide Prevention LifeLine.[40]

For the reader to better appreciate the power of SGRP as a viable method for training a large group of clinicians in complex interview strategies, it is valuable to provide a brief overview of the CASE Approach itself. Before doing so, three educational terms from the specialty of clinical interviewing can serve as lenses for our exploration. (1) An "interviewing principle" is a guiding concept for approaching an interviewing task. Interviewing principles are abstractions that suggest why an interview technique or strategy is being used and when to use it. For instance, an interviewing principle might be: before asking a question about a sensitive or taboo topic, such as suicide, say something that metacommunicates to the patient that it is safe to share information about the topic in question. (2) By contrast, an "interviewing technique" (the real-world application of an interviewing principle) is a behaviorally specific set of words (often a single statement or a single question) that has been operationalized and tagged with a name. Thus, the aforementioned interviewing principle can be employed by using either of two specific interviewing techniques: normalization and shame attenuation, of which an example of shame attenuation would be, "With all of the pain of your divorce, have you been having any thoughts of killing yourself?" (3) An interviewing strategy is the sequential use of two or more interviewing techniques to address a complex interviewing task. The CASE Approach is a sophisticated interviewing strategy for uncovering suicidal ideation.

More specifically, the CASE Approach is a flexible and practical interview strategy for eliciting suicidal ideation, planning, behaviors, and intent designed to help the interviewer explore both the inner pains of the client and the suicidal planning that often reflects these pains. It was designed to increase validity, decrease errors of omission, and increase the client's sense of safety with the interviewer while discussing intimate details regarding actual suicidal ideation, intent, and behaviors. In the CASE Approach, clinicians are trained to flexibly uncover suicidal ideation and intent using a sophisticated set of questions and interview strategies, as opposed to asking a simplistic set of rote questions on the mere presence of suicidal plans. The techniques and strategies of the CASE Approach are concretely behaviorally defined; consequently, it can be taught readily and the skill level of the clinician tested easily, and documented for quality assurance purposes individually (via macrotraining) and within a group format (via SGRP).

In the CASE Approach, the interviewer explores the suicidal feelings, ideation, plans, intent, and actions of the client over four contiguous time regions, hence its name. First, the clinician begins by sensitively and carefully exploring the client's presenting suicidal ideation/actions if present, a period of time that generally includes the last 48 hours but can go back a week or two as deemed necessary (Region #1 Presenting Suicide Events). Second, the clinician explores the client's suicidal ideation/actions during the previous two months (Region #2 Recent Suicide Events). After completing this exploration, Region #3 (Past Suicide Events), consisting of the past suicide attempts, is explored. Finally, the clinician explores Region #4 (Immediate Suicide Events) consisting of suicidal feelings, ideation, and intent that arise during the interview itself, and the client's views on possible future suicidal thoughts and what to do if they arise (**Fig. 1**).

A hallmark of the CASE Approach is the flexible use of seven specific interviewing techniques, designed to increase the validity of the elicited data, while exploring each of the four chronological regions described. These seven validity techniques (normalization, shame attenuation, the behavioral incident, gentle assumption, denial of the specific, the catch-all question, and symptom amplification) were culled from the preexisting clinical interviewing literature in the fields of counseling, clinical psychology, and psychiatry.

Limitations of space prevent a detailed description of the CASE Approach here (appropriate resources for a complete review of the approach are provided later), but I want to share enough of the strategy that the reader can grasp how SGRP can be effectively utilized to train clinicians in its use. To accomplish this process, let us look at one of the validity techniques used in the CASE Approach, "the behavioral incident," and how it is used in Region #1 of the CASE Approach (eliciting suicidal ideation, intent, and behaviors in the last 48 hours).

"Behavioral incidents," an interviewing technique originally described by the clinical psychologist Pascal,[23] are questions that ask for specific facts, behavioral details, or trains of thought, as with, "How many pills did you take?", "Did you load the gun?," or "What stopped you from jumping?," or which simply ask the patient to describe what happened sequentially, as with, "What did you do next?" Thus there are two types of behavioral incidents: (1) fact-finding behavioral incidents and (2) sequencing behavioral incidents. By using a series of behavioral incidents sequentially, the interviewer can create an interviewing strategy that can sometimes help a patient to enhance validity by recreating, step by step, the unfolding of a potentially taboo topic such as a suicide attempt or an act of domestic violence.

In this interview strategy, during the exploration of Region #1 (The Presenting Event), the interviewer asks the patient to describe the suicide attempt from beginning to end. During this description the clinician gently, but persistently, utilizes a series of behavioral incidents guiding the patient to create a "verbal video" of the attempt step by step. Readers familiar with cognitive-behavioral therapy (CBT) will recognize this strategy as one of the cornerstone assessment tools of CBT—a "behavioral analysis."

If an important piece of the account is missing, the clinician returns to that area, exploring with a series of clarifying behavioral incidents, until the clinician feels confident that he or she has an accurate picture of what happened. This serial use of behavioral incidents not only increases the clinician's understanding of the extent of the patient's intent and actions, it also decreases any unwarranted assumptions by the clinician that may distort the database. Creating such a verbal video, the clinician

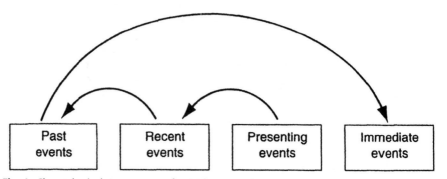

Fig. 1. Chronological Assessment of Suicide Events (CASE Approach).

will frequently uncover a more accurate picture of the suicidal behavior and the suicidal intent it may reflect in a naturally unfolding conversational mode.

In this fashion the clinician can feel more confident of delineating an accurate picture of how close the patient actually came to attempting suicide. The resulting scenario may prove to be radically different and more suggestive of imminent danger from what would have been relayed by the patient if the interviewer had merely asked an opinion of the client such as, "Did you come close to actually using the gun?," to which an embarrassed or cagey patient might quickly reply, "Oh no, not really."

Perhaps one of the most sophisticated uses of the validity techniques occurs in Region #2 of the CASE Approach (Recent Suicide Events, including suicidal thoughts, plans, and behaviors over the past 2 months). In this region of the CASE Approach, five of the validity techniques, namely the behavioral incident (BI), gentle assumption (GA), denial of the specific (DS), the catch-all question (CAQ), and symptom amplification (SA), are flexibly interwoven to uncover hidden suicidal intent and behaviors, with a special emphasis on uncovering the suicidal method of choice in a patient hesitant to share his or her true method of choice and severity of intent (**Fig. 2**).

Without knowledge of the definitions and uses of all the validity techniques, **Fig. 2** may not make a lot of sense, but all the reader needs to glean from it, for our purposes, is the fact that this exploration uses a complex series of interviewing sequences (strategies) composed of well-defined interviewing techniques. Despite its complexity, most participants being trained via SGRP can learn this sequence and behaviorally perform most, if not all, of it at the end of the training session in a reasonable manner without any cue sheets.

Many options exist for the reader to learn more about the CASE Approach. For an up-to-date article I recommend the two-part article on the CASE Approach, which is available as a free pdf at the homepage of the Training Institute for Suicide assessment and Clinical Interviewing (TISA).[29,30] If you prefer a book chapter, the recent chapter entitled "The Interpersonal Art of Suicide Assessment: Interviewing Techniques for Uncovering Suicidal Intent, Ideation, and Actions" from *The American Psychiatric Publishing Textbook of Suicide Assessment and Management*, 2nd Edition, is devoted entirely to the CASE Approach and is an excellent resource.[15] To understand how the CASE Approach can be integrated with other critical aspects of performing an effective suicide assessment including the judicious use of risk/protective factors, practical approaches to the clinical formulation of risk, and principles for soundly documenting risk from clinical and forensic perspectives, the reader is referred to the book *The Practical Art of Suicide Assessment: A Guide for Mental Health Professionals and Substance Abuse Counselors.*[32]

Having briefly explored both the utility of the CASE Approach and some of its clinical nuances, it should be easy to imagine its potential clinical and educational value. At the same time one can envision the challenge of teaching such a complex interviewing strategy to a reasonable degree of fidelity with a large number of graduate students or medical/nursing students, or to hospital staff. Moreover, as noted earlier, whatever learning approach the graduate school, residency, or institute would choose to use, the approach would need to be both enjoyable and effective for trainees to realistically gain from it, a characteristic that historically has proved to be elusive with group role-playing formats.

In this regard, before describing how to perform SGRP, it seems requisite to provide data that lend some support to the idea that SGRP may have the power to accomplish the aforementioned task. Such an advance would open the door for educators to ensure that entire graduate school classes in mental health disciplines or entire medical and nursing school classes could be effectively trained to elicit suicidal ideation

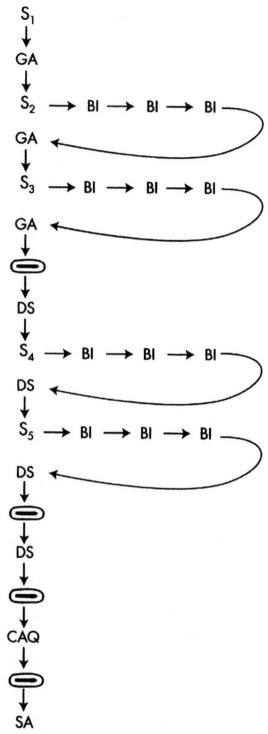

Fig. 2. Prototypic exploration of the region of recent suicide events. The schema should be flexibly adapted in response to clients' answers and clinical presentation. BI, behavioral incident; CAQ, catch-all question; DS, denial of the specific; GA, gentle assumption; S, suicide method; SA, symptom amplification. Bar within ellipse indicates client denial of suicidal ideation.

and intent in an effective fashion. Such a sweeping educational accomplishment could potentially save many lives.

A participant satisfaction study on scripted group role-playing

At the TISA (www.suicideassessment.com), initial development and subsequent refinement of SGRP has been ongoing for over 15 years. TISA has been providing formal certification in the CASE Approach to mental health professionals for more than 5 years. For the purposes of improving design, an early internal quality assurance study was undertaken of 20 consecutive SGRP trainings with varying degrees of participant size ranging from 8 to 28. The study was not done under strict research protocols, and is presented as a seed study, with all of the typical limitations of seed research. For instance, accurate records of percent participant evaluation return were not kept, although it is estimated that an 85% or higher evaluation return was achieved. (Note that subsequent to this study, TISA has been providing Level 1 Certification Trainings on the CASE Approach in which *certification is not granted unless the participant returns a completed evaluation form*. Only 2 evaluations have not been accounted for in 19 trainings. The results in the evaluation scores show no apparent differences from the results found in the original quality assurance study whose results are reported below.)

The SGRP format is described in detail in the last section of this article. It was developed in answer to the provocative question, "How would role-playing be experienced by participants if there was little or no acting involved?" Consequently the most striking innovation in SGRP is the use of scripted role-playing. In SGRP all role-plays are scripted, with little or no need for acting, which greatly decreases participant fears of role-playing while increasing both efficiency of practice and ability to consolidate techniques effectively. Because all of the role-plays are designed by the training team, each role-play creates an ideal opportunity for the clinician attempting to master the given interviewing technique or strategy to practice it. In addition, as the role-plays are designed by the training team, they efficiently address each learning skill and eliminate wasted time by "overacting" participants.

Each validity technique and its use in the CASE Approach is practiced in pods of four, participants (referred to during training as A, B, C, and D) actively coached by the trainer(s) and fellow participants in each of the four-person practice pods. Didactic training and video illustration is provided on all four regions of the CASE Approach. Intensive experiential training using SGRP is done on Region #1 (Presenting Events) and Region #2 (Recent Events), a process that is the focus of more than 90% of the day. By the end of the day, many of the participants have been able to behaviorally demonstrate, without any written cues, the ability to perform both of these complex regions of the CASE Approach in a reasonably sensitive and comprehensive fashion.

Generally speaking, of the 28 trainees there might be 1 to 3 who struggle somewhat during the day but can still replicate about 30% of the strategy. Despite their struggles with the more complex aspects of the CASE Approach (such as Region #2 concerning recent suicide events over the past 2 months), these trainees achieve by the end of the day an effective ability to raise the topic of suicide sensitively and to subsequently explore, by creating a verbal video with behavioral incidents, the extent of the patient's action taken on the presenting method. By contrast, most of the trainees can reasonably reproduce, without cues, the techniques and strategies of the first two regions of the CASE Approach including the complex interview sequences of Region #2 (see **Fig. 2**). In a group of 28 participants there are, remarkably, usually a handful of trainees who can demonstrate even the most complex sequences of Region #2 to complete fidelity without cues.

The 20 trainings comprising the study (with a combined cohort of 427) promptly began at 8:30 AM and ended at 5:00 PM, with a minimum of 6.5 hours of actual training time. The remaining time was allotted to lunch and periodic brief breaks. Consisting primarily of role-playing, interspersed with small segments of didactic training and video demonstrations, such full-day role-play trainings were rigorous and demanding to say the least.

Participants were asked to respond to the following 5-point Likert Scale statement by rating it from 0 (disagree) to 4 (agree): "The content of the training provided useful information for my clinical work."

The average response to this statement was a 3.9 across all disciplines including licensed clinical social workers (LCSWs), nurses, psychiatrists, psychologists, therapists, counselors, and other mental health professionals (see **Figs. 1** and **2**). This highly positive response supports the belief that the CASE Approach, as taught via SGRP, provides innovative interviewing techniques for uncovering suicidal ideation and intent that are valued by participants ranging from the least experienced (graduate students) to the most experienced with many years of experience behind them.

For instance, in this cohort of 427, 99 of the clinicians reported having been in clinical practice for more than 20 years (ranging from 20 to 45 years postgraduate training). These experienced clinicians also rated the above statement at 3.9, reflecting that the CASE Approach contains new material not encountered in previous continuing education regarding suicide assessment. It is rare to find experienced clinicians responding to a full day's training on suicide assessment with such enthusiasm and even rarer when they are asked to perform role-playing throughout the day.

In addition, participants were asked to rate the following 5-point (0–4) Likert Scale statement: "I would recommend this training to a fellow colleague."

A total of 427 participants responded (**Figs. 3** and **4**). The average response to the above statement was once again 3.9 across all participants. There was no

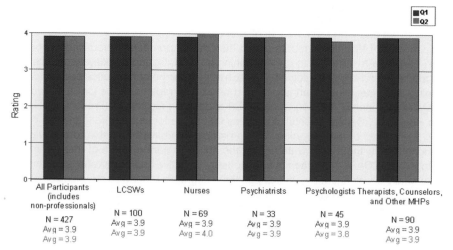

Fig. 3. By professional discipline, average participant rating for scripted group role-playing (SGRP) on the chronological assessment of suicide events (CASE Approach). Results in blue are the average of the trainees' responses to Question #1: "The content of the training provided useful information for my clinical work" rated from 0 (disagree) to 4 (agree). Results in red are the average of the trainees' responses to Question #2: "I would recommend this training to a fellow colleague" rated from 0 (disagree) to 4 (agree). (Compiled from 20 consecutive trainings using SGRP, April 22, 2012, Shawn Christopher Shea, MD.)

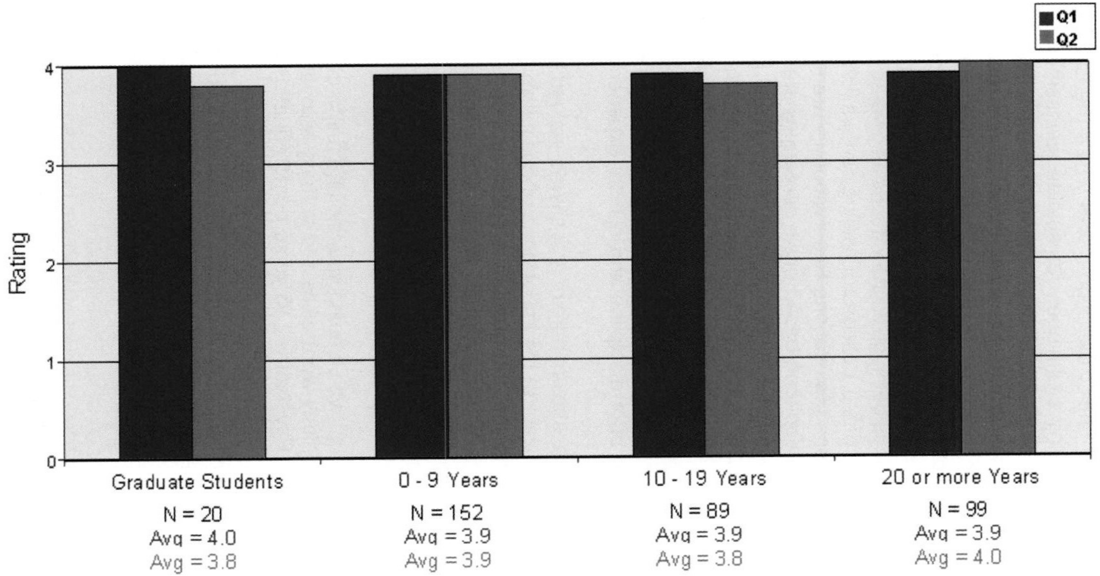

Fig. 4. By years of clinical experience, average participant rating for scripted group role-playing (SGRP) on the chronological assessment of suicide events (CASE Approach). Results in blue are the average of the trainees' responses to Question #1: "The content of the training provided useful information for my clinical work" rated from 0 (disagree) to 4 (agree). Results in red are the average of the trainees' responses to Question #2: "I would recommend this training to a fellow colleague" rated from 0 (disagree) to 4 (agree). (Compiled from 20 consecutive trainings using SGRP, April 22, 2012, Shawn Christopher Shea, MD.)

significant difference in this average across all disciplines including LCSWs, nurses, psychiatrists, psychologists, therapists, counselors, and other mental health professionals. Once again there was no difference among various groups delineated by years of experience.

This satisfaction rating is a high one in any training, but is remarkably high for a full-day training based primarily on role-playing. It demonstrates the power of SGRP to make skill-enhancing role-playing psychologically safe and enjoyable.

The surprising results seem to reflect the degree with which the CASE Approach itself is providing new interviewing techniques for suicide assessment, which are believed to be both novel and of practical use to even experienced clinicians. Of more immediate relevance to this article, however, these results mean that SGRP has created a role-playing environment that feels safe, sophisticated, and comfortable for participants across all disciplines and across all levels of experience.

Moreover, in this cohort of 20 different trainings, SGRP demonstrated robust generalizability to different clinical settings being given in locations as diverse as hospitals (El Camino Hospital, El Camino, California), college counseling centers (University of Oregon), Native American reservations (Six Nations Reservation in Brantford, Canada), VAs (Fort Wayne, Indiana) and telephone-based crisis centers where role-playing is done back-to-back in SGRP to simulate telephone intervention (West Bend, Indiana).

Another striking feature of SGRP is the fact that participants across all disciplines (including nonprofessionals such as volunteers at crisis lines for suicide prevention) and participants ranging across all levels of experience (from graduate students to clinicians with more than 40 years of experience) *can be taught in the same class.* Indeed this cross-fertilization, in both discipline and clinical experience, seemed to enhance learning and enjoyment.

As trainers, empirical data as shown herein are always valued. In addition, I feel trainers are particularly cognizant of the importance of qualitative data from participants as well. As one can imagine, the qualitative comments on SGRP in all examples of its use have been particularly robust. As an illustration, I now share a small sample of comments from the last SGRP performed before the writing of this article in which participants commented specifically about their experience of the role-playing:

> "Usually not a fan of role-play, but with it being specific and reinforcing the interviewing techniques, it was definitely worthwhile and actually enjoyable."
> —Psychiatrist, 15 years postgraduation experience

> "The scripted role-play is a brilliant idea. It ensures that all are involved utilizing the skill set taught. The CASE Approach has made me more confident in my interview skills."
> —Nurse, 6 years postgraduation experience

> "This would be an excellent graduate course. Wish we had had more hands-on practice like this. Scripted role-play felt very comfortable, and I am someone who will avoid role-plays at all costs."
> —Social worker, LCSW-A, first year postgraduation

> "Practical information presented. Really enjoyed role-play, and I typically HATE role-plays." (Note that besides being printed in all CAPS, the word "hate" was double underlined.)
> —Licensed professional counselor, 12 years postgraduation

Format and principles of scripted group role-playing
To illustrate the principles and format of SGRP, I now describe its use in teaching the CASE Approach. SGRP can be used to teach any interviewing technique or strategy (uncovering incest/domestic violence, uncovering substance use, performing a sensitive differential diagnosis). It is used, to its best capabilities, when one is teaching behaviorally specific and operationalized interviewing techniques and/or interviewing strategies that are composed of specific sequences of recommended techniques as seen with the CASE Approach.

Structure of the training pods and flow At one end of the room, a didactic teaching section is created where all didactic instruction is performed (occupying only about one-fifth of the room's area). Behind the rows of chairs the pods are arranged in the remaining four-fifths of the room consisting of groups of 4 participants each, allowing ample room between pods to decrease noise, for all pods are simultaneously active during role-playing.

Each participant receives a packet of role-plays indicating a pod number and a designation as to their position in the pod (A, B, C, D). Each individual interviewing technique (behavioral incident, gentle assumption, and so forth) that is used in the CASE Approach is always didactically taught, and subsequently the participants move to their respective pods to experientially practice the technique directly after the didactics of each technique. Later in the day, as interviewing techniques are sequenced into interview strategies such as uncovering Region #1 (Presenting Suicide Events) and Region #2 (Recent Suicide Events) of the CASE Approach, each region will be practiced within a pod, providing the chance to learn the new sequence but to also consolidate any previously learned interviewing techniques, for they are repeatedly used in the interview sequences.

When beginning a pod module regarding a single specific interviewing technique (such as normalization, shame attenuation, gentle assumption) or an interview strategy (such as creating a verbal video with a sequence of behavioral incidents), the trainer asks all "A's" to pick up their role-play folders: they will play the patient. The "B's" will practice the interviewing technique (such as normalization, shame attenuation) or interview strategy (such as creating a verbal video with behavioral incidents). The "C's" and "D's" will function as coaches, immediately providing feedback after the interviewing technique or strategy has been practiced. With SGRP, the coaching provided by the trainers is significantly enhanced by the coaching feedback given from participants to each other. I have been impressed by the quality of participant-to-participant feedback in SGRP. As the 7 pods of 4 are practicing, the trainer circulates about the room from pod to pod providing constructive feedback and modeling as needed (note that SGRP can be done with a total group number ranging from 4 to 28; a number larger than 28 is not recommended as it dilutes the coaching time from the trainer). While the trainer provides feedback to one pod, the other pods continue their work. After the first run-through of the technique and after the coaching has been provided by participants C and D, the participant coaches ask the role-play to be repeated several times so as to consolidate the interviewer's acquisition of the new technique or strategy being practiced.

After all groups have performed these tasks, the trainer asks all "B's" to pick up their role-play folders: they will play the patient. The "A's" now practice the specific technique (normalization, shame attenuation, gentle assumption, and so forth) or strategy (eg, verbal video). "C's" and "D's" coach yet again. Note that the act of coaching is a learning experience itself, for the coaches must process the concept of the technique or strategy in a sophisticated manner to provide feedback.

After all groups have performed these tasks, the trainer asks all "C's" to pick up their role-play folders: they will play the patient. The "D's" now practice the specific technique (eg, normalization) or strategy (eg, verbal video). The "A's" and "B's" now coach. Note that these coaches are slightly more seasoned, for they have each had a chance to practice the technique or strategy and they have both experienced being a patient with whom the technique or strategy is being utilized when they played the patient role. Consequently, these coaches may provide an even more sophisticated level of feedback.

After all groups have performed these tasks, the trainer asks all "D's" to pick up their role-play folders: they will play the patient. The "C's" now practice the specific technique (normalization) or strategy (verbal video). The "A's" and "B's" coach yet again.

Before each role-play begins, the participants playing the role are given 2 to 3 minutes to read through the role-play. This quiet time allows them a chance to note their directions and to become comfortable with what they will read directly. There are also written cues of what content must be included if they are providing a sentence or two of "more spontaneous dialogue."

When designing your role-plays for A through D, it is important to purposefully design each role-play to demonstrate for the pod a specific nuance of the interview technique or strategy that is being practiced. For instance, when creating role-plays A through D for practicing the making of a verbal video, the designer may make "A" a role-play regarding an overdose, "B" a role-play on the use of a gun, "C" a role-play on hanging, and "D" a role-play on jumping from a bridge or building. Thus, with every role-play each member of the pod is learning a new nuance about the technique or strategy being used.

As the day proceeds, once the specific techniques that are to be used in a more complex interviewing strategy have been practiced, the training moves on to practicing the more complex interviewing strategies. In short, as the day proceeds the role-plays become more and more complex as one moves from practicing interviewing techniques to practicing interviewing strategies such as exploring Region #1 or Region #2 of the CASE Approach.

At no time should interviewers have anything on their laps. Cue sheets or "cheat sheets" are not allowed, as they slow skill acquisition.

Core principles for designing scripted group role-plays Historically the term "scripted role-playing" has been used to describe a variety of formats. It is sometimes used not as a method of skills enhancement role-playing but as a platform for group discussion, as has been described by Schweickert and Heeren[41] when teaching sexual history taking. In this format, a scenario in which the words of both the patient and the clinician are completely written is used. The role-play is then read by two participants for use as a platform for group discussion. Although this is an excellent and creative method for generating group discussion, in such a format there is no chance for participants to actually practice interviewing techniques.

In the group format of skill enhancement whereby participants are expected to receive a chance to experientially practice interviewing techniques, "scripted role-playing" generally means that the participant playing the patient has been given written instructions on who he or she is playing, characteristics of the patient, and possible symptoms, stresses, and so forth. Occasionally these scripts include some specific statements that the "patient" should say. As the role-play is begun, the other participant then practices his or her interviewing skills.

SGRP is a significantly more advanced form of scripted role-playing. Acting is essentially removed or greatly minimized, which I have found markedly decreases participant anxiety, eliminates problems with participants overacting, and enhances the focus of the role-plays. All role-playing of patients is done by the participants in the training pods, not by the trainer.

In SGRP all role-plays begin with a cue statement *read* by the role-player from his or her script. This initiating statement is designed to create the best possible cue for the participant learning the technique to practice it. *In addition, before the role-play begins, the trainer reads the cue statement aloud to the entire set of participants and states the exact words of the interviewing technique that the interviewer is to use.* This simple and immediate modeling of the interviewing technique being practiced markedly increases the likelihood of the interviewer succeeding, both consolidating the technique and creating a positive sense of gained expertise. The trainer then tells the role-players to read their cue statements and the role-playing begins. As soon as the interviewing technique is done, the role-play is stopped by the coaches and feedback is provided by the participant coaches in the learning pod.

When the role-play involves practicing a more complex interview strategy composed of a sequence of interview techniques (such as practicing making a verbal video of the extent of action taken on a suicide attempt), *a hallmark of SGRP is the fact that specific, sometimes detailed, instructions are given in the written role-player sheet as to when to say what and how to say it, so as to maximize the learning experience for the participant practicing the interview strategy*. Appendices 1 and 2 present examples of scripted role-plays.

SUMMARY

Hopefully, this article provides a useful introduction to the art of role-playing in both the individual format and group format using SGRP. There is little doubt that role-playing can provide powerful learning opportunities, but to do so it must be done well. The purpose of this article is to impart some guidance toward this goal.

Of particular importance has been the opportunity in this revised article to introduce the concept of SGRP. The potential promise of this educational advancement in the format of group role-playing (allowing large groups of trainees to practice and master complex interviewing skills in a reasonable amount of time) is tangible and within reach. SGRP may greatly enhance and assure the acquisition of critical complex interviewing skills in health care providers across all disciplines, an educational goal that has not been achievable to date. SGRP can be used to train skills in a variety of tasks such as uncovering incest/domestic violence, uncovering substance abuse, achieving improved competence in crisis intervention skills, performing a sensitive differential diagnosis, and, of course, suicide assessment.

Regarding the latter skill set, the promise of SGRP, as a tool to concretely reduce the suicide rate, is particularly exciting. As mentioned earlier, it is well documented that at least 50% of patients who kill themselves have seen a primary care clinician within 1 month of their deaths.[26] A typical primary care clinician is seeing patients who warrant a suicide assessment on a daily basis. To prepare medical, nursing, physician assistant, and clinical pharmacy students for this future task, as part of the numerous competency skills they are required to demonstrate before graduation, every student could be required by their faculty to participate in a single-day training in the CASE Approach using SGRP. Acquiring this skill would require only a single day of training in the course of a 4-year program.

If such training resulted in only 50% of these students subsequently effectively uncovering suicidal ideation in their subsequent careers, and if such improved delineation resulted in preventing a subsequent suicide in only 50% of the times it was used, the suicide rate could, theoretically, be reduced by 12.5% across the country. This type of model has been successfully used on a national level in emergency medicine and nursing, where a full day of coached training and certification is required in Advanced Cardio Life Support (ACLS), with the subsequent saving of many lives over the following decades.

Obviously such training would also be of immediate use in the education of psychiatric residents and nurses, in addition to graduate students across all mental health disciplines. Although the research on SGRP is in an early stage of development, the hope it represents is indeed tangibly exciting.

REFERENCES

1. The 360 degree view: a question of competence. Rochester Medicine 2006;26.
2. Ivey A. Microcounseling: innovations in interviewer training. Springfield (MO): Charles C. Thomas; 1971.
3. Daniels T. Microcounselling research: what 450 data-based studies reveal. In: Ivey A, Ivey M, editors. Intentional interviewing and counseling. Belmont (CA): Wadsworth Publishing; 2003. Interactive CD-ROM.
4. Shea SC, Barney C. Macrotraining: a "how-to" primer for using serial role-playing to train complex clinical interviewing tasks such as suicide assessment. Psychiatr Clin North Am 2007;30:e1–29.
5. Becking D, Berkel T, Betermieux S, et al. Altering the roles of learners and tutors in a virtual practical training by means of role-playing. In: Lassner D, McNaught C, editors. Proceedings of World Conference on Educational Multimedia, Hypermedia and Telecommunications. Chesapeake (VA): AACE; 2003. p. 2278–81.
6. Phelps CL, Willcockson I. The LEARN curriculum: hands-on classroom experiments. New York: Society for Neuroscience Abstract Viewer & Itinerary Planner; 2002 [abstract: 22.42].
7. Smith RC, Lyles JS, Mettler J, et al. The effectiveness of intensive training for residents in interviewing: a randomized, controlled study. Ann Intern Med 1998; 128(2):118–26.
8. Baker DP, Gustafson S, Beaubien JM, et al. Medical team training programs in health care. Advances in Patient Safety 2005;4:253–67.
9. Barach PR, Mohr JJ. Microsystems simulation: designing and evaluating an approach to patient safety and systems thinking. Abstract A:1108. Presented at the Anesthesiology Abstracts of Scientific Papers Annual Meeting. 2002.
10. Knowles C, Kinchington F, Erwin J, et al. A randomized controlled trial of the effectiveness of combining video role play with traditional methods of delivering undergraduate medical education. Sex Transm Infect 2001;77:376–80.
11. Jeffries PR. A framework for designing, implementing, and evaluating simulations used as teaching strategies in nursing. Nurs Educ Perspect 2005;26(2): 96–103.
12. Deveugele M, Derese A, De Maesschalck S, et al. Teaching communication skills to medical students, a challenge in the curriculum? Patient Educ Couns 2005; 58(3):265–70.
13. Scisson EH. Counseling for results: principles and practice of helping professions. Pacific Grove (CA): Brooks/Cole; 1993.
14. Daniels T. Microcounseling research: what over 450 data-based studies reveal. In: Ivey A, Ivey M, editors. Intentional interviewing and counseling, Interactive CD-ROM. Pacific Grove, CA: Brooks Cole Publishing Co.; 2003. p. 15.

15. Shea SC. The interpersonal art of suicide assessment: interviewing techniques for uncovering suicidal intent, ideation, and actions. In: Simon RI, Hales RE, editors. The American psychiatric publishing textbook of suicide assessment and management. 2nd edition. Washington, DC: American Psychiatric Publishing; 2012. p. 29–56.
16. Shea SC, Director. Training Institute for Suicide Assessment and Clinical Interviewing. Available at: www.suicideassessment.com. Accessed January 06, 2015.
17. Harden RM, Stevenson M, Downie WW, et al. Assessment of clinical competence using objective structured clinical examination. Br Med J 1975;1(5955): 447–51.
18. Shea SC, Barney C. Facilic supervision and schematics: the art of training psychiatric residents and other mental health professionals how to structure clinical interviews sensitively. Psychiatr Clin North Am 2007;30:e51–96.
19. Shea SC. Psychiatric interviewing: the art of understanding–a practical guide for psychiatrists, psychologists, counselors, social workers, nurses, and other mental health professionals. 2nd edition. Philadelphia: W.B. Saunders Company; 1998.
20. Benedek EP. Interpersonal process recall: an innovative technique. J Med Educ 1977;52:939–41.
21. Pryor K. Don't shoot the dog—the new art of teaching and training. Revised edition. Bantam Books; 1999.
22. Shea SC. Macrotraining manual. Training Institute for Suicide Assessment and Clinical Interviewing (TISA). Copyright 1997.
23. Pascal GR. The practical art of diagnostic interviewing. Homewood (IL): Dow-Jones-Irwin; 1983.
24. Pomeroy WB, Flax CC, Wheeler CC. Taking a sex history. New York: The Free Press; 1982.
25. Shea SC. Improving medication adherence: how to talk with patients about their medications. Philadelphia: Lippincott Williams & Wilkins; 2006.
26. Luoma JB, Martin CE, Pearson JL. Contact with mental health and primary care providers before suicide: a review of the evidence. Am J Psychiatry 2002;159: 909–16.
27. Shea SC. The chronological assessment of suicide events: a practical interviewing strategy for the elicitation of suicidal ideation. J Clin Psychiatry 1998;59(Suppl 20):58–72.
28. Reed M, Shea SC. Suicide assessment in college students: innovations in uncovering suicidal ideation and intent (CASE Approach). In: Lamis DA, Lester D, editors. Understanding and preventing college student suicide. Springfield (IL): Charles. C. Thomas Publisher, Ltd; 2011. p. 197–222.
29. Shea SC. Suicide assessment: part 1—uncovering suicidal intent, a sophisticated art. Psychiatric Times 2009;26(12):17–9. Available at: http://www.PsychiatricTimes. com. Accessed May 9, 2011.
30. Shea SC. Suicide assessment: part 2—uncovering suicidal intent, using the chronological assessment of suicidal events (CASE Approach). 2009. Available at: http://www.PsychiatricTimes.com. Accessed May 9, 2011.
31. Knoll, J. Correctional suicide risk assessment and prevention. Correctional Mental Health Report: Practice, Administration, Law 10(5):65–80, 2009.
32. Shea SC. The practical art of suicide assessment: a guide for mental health professionals and substance abuse counselors. Stoddard (NH): Mental Health Presses; 2011.
33. Shea SC. The delicate art of eliciting suicidal ideation. Psychiatr Ann 2004;34: 385–400.

34. Shea SC. Practical tips for eliciting suicidal ideation for the substance abuse professional. Counselor, the Magazine for Addiction Professionals 2001;2: 14–24.
35. Shea SC. The chronological assessment of suicide events (the CASE Approach): an introduction for the front-line clinician. NewsLink (Newsletter of the American Association of Suicidology) 2002;29:12–3.
36. Shea SC. Tips for uncovering suicidal ideation in the primary care setting. Part of the 4-part CD-ROM series titled hidden diagnosis: uncovering anxiety and depressive disorders (version 2.0). Philadelphia: GlaxoSmithKline; 1999.
37. Shea SC. The chronological assessment of suicide events: an innovative method for training residents to competently elicit suicidal ideation. Presented at the American Association of Directors of Psychiatric Residency Training (AADPRT). Puerto Rico, March 6–9, 2003.
38. Shea SC. Innovations in uncovering suicidal ideation with vets and soldiers: the chronological assessment of suicide events (CASE Approach). Presented at the Department of Defense/Veterans Administration Annual Suicide Prevention Conference. San Antonio, TX, January 12–15, 2009.
39. Shea SC. Innovations in eliciting suicidal ideation: the chronological assessment of suicide events (CASE Approach). Presented at: the Annual Meetings of the American Association of Suicidology from 1999 through 2014.
40. Shea SC. The Chronological assessment of suicide events (CASE Approach) as taught via scripted group role-playing (SGRP) for telephone crisis line providers. Presented at the Annual Meeting of LIfeLine. Washington, DC, 2009.
41. Schweickert EA, Hereen AB. Scripted role play: a technique for teaching sexual history taking. J Am Osteopath Assoc 1999;99(5):275–6.

APPENDIX 1: SAMPLE ROLE-PLAY SCRIPT FOR A SINGLE INTERVIEWING TECHNIQUE

Note to Reader: The following is an example of a role-play script for use by all the seven "A" trainees in the seven pods (if there are 28 participants split into seven groups of four each) when introducing "gentle assumption". Remember that you would need to create a unique role-play script for each of the B, C, and D participants for use when it is their turn to play the patient in the pod exercise devoted to practicing gentle assumption. You would design each role-play for the A, B, C, and D participants to illustrate a slightly different aspect of using a gentle assumption. Thus with each role-play something new about the use of gentle assumptions is learned by every member of the pod.

In a more generic sense, Appendix 1 is provided as a model to be used in designing role-plays that you create to consolidate a previously practiced interviewing technique while simultaneously teaching a new interviewing technique. In the following role-play script the interviewer must once again use a "shame attenuation" (first introduced as an interviewing technique in the immediately preceding role-play and now consolidated in this role-play through repetition). The interviewer must then use a series of "gentle assumptions" (a technique that is being introduced in this role-play for the very first time). Thus you can see the fashion in which serial repetition from role-play to role-play is often used in SGRP to simultaneously consolidate previously practiced interviewing techniques while introducing a new interviewing technique.

Note that key directions for the role-player are often printed in bold and/or ALL CAPS so as to "jump off the page" ensuring that the role player can quickly see what he or she is to do next in the role-play. Occasionally, italics are also utilized to emphasize points of protocol.

Gentle Assumption for Role-Player A

Consolidation exercise for Shame Attenuation and new acquisition RP for Gentle Assumption

Who you are: For the sake of getting into the role a bit, here is some background.

You are a 22-year-old who has developed a major depression triggered by a break-up with your boyfriend/girlfriend with whom you have had a long-standing rocky relationship. (This material will be shared by the trainer with the whole group before the role-play begins, for it represents the information garnered by the interviewer in the first 15 minutes of the interview.)

Your first response:

After the interviewer uses a shame attenuation (eg, "With all of your pain, have you been having any thoughts of killing yourself?") you will say **"yes."**

After the interviewer asks, "What have you thought of doing?" You will say, **"Hanging myself."**

After each subsequent gentle assumption by the interviewer, give **one** of the following methods starting at the top straight down.

When the list is done, after the interviewer uses a gentle assumption simply say, "No other ways" and the drill will be done:

1. Driving my car into a tree

2. Jumping off a bridge

3. Overdosing on aspirin

4. Shooting myself

5. Cutting myself

Tips for Role-Player:

1. Provide each method **ONLY** after the clinician uses a gentle assumption.

2. If clinician **does not** use a gentle assumption (eg, asks something like, "Have you thought of other ways of killing yourself?")

ANSWER WITH A SIMPLE *"NO."*

Cue Statement to Begin Role-Play: Just say, **"I don't know what I'm going to do now. I don't know if it's worth going on without him/her. I just don't know."** (Interviewer will follow up with a shame attenuation.)

APPENDIX 2: SAMPLE ROLE-PLAY SCRIPT FOR A TEACHING A COMPLEX INTERVIEWING STRATEGY SUCH AS REGION #2 IN THE CASE APPROACH

Note to Reader: The following is an example of a role-play script for use by all the seven "A" trainees in the seven pods (if there are 28 participants split into seven groups of four each) when introducing the exploration of Region #2 in the CASE Approach (Recent Suicide Events over the past two months). Remember that you would need to create a unique role-play script for each of the B, C, and D participants for use when it is their turn to play the patient in the pod exercise devoted to practicing the exploration of Region #2 (Recent Suicide Events). You would design each role-play for the A, B, C, and D participants to illustrate a slightly different aspect of the exploration of Recent Suicide Events (differing suicide methods, differing number of methods considered, different method of choice etc.). To do so, you would need to create a completely different patient for participants A, B, C, and D to play. Thus with each role-play script something new about the exploration of Recent Suicide Events is learned by every member of the pod.

Script for Role-player A: Exploration of Recent Events (Past 2 Months)

1. **Who you are (What has been uncovered in the first 15 minutes of interview):**

   You are a 37-year-old newspaper reporter who has just lost his job because his/her newspaper has folded in the harsh economic times. You are also heavily stressed by fears that your spouse is having an affair. *(This will be read by the trainer to the whole group before role-play begins.)*

2. **What has already been uncovered during "verbal video" of Presenting Event:**

   When exploring the Presenting Region of the CASE Approach, the clinician uncovered that, about 1 week ago, you had gone to a bridge, got up to the rail, but stopped. Looked briefly over the rail and quickly went away.

Cue Statement for Beginning the Role-Play: "I couldn't jump. I just couldn't do that to my kids, but sometimes I wonder if they wouldn't be better with me dead. The only thing I'm really good at is writing copy, and newspapers are a thing of the past."

Script:

Clinician will make bridging question about jumping thoughts over past 2 months

   You will say "No."

Clinician will use Gentle Assumption

   You will say, "I've thought of overdosing."

<u>GRADUALLY</u> SHARE THE FOLLOWING AS THE CLINICIAN MAKES A VERBAL VIDEO USING BEHAVIORAL INCIDENTS

   1. **Bought some aspirin a several weeks ago**
   2. **Went home (your wife was out with some friends) and drank a 6-pack of beer in your recreation room in your basement**
   3. **Proceeded to put about 20 pills in your hand**
   4. **Only took about 10 pills**
   5. **Once again, couldn't do it because of your kids**

Clinician will use Gentle Assumption

   You will say, "Nothing really."

Clinician will use Denials of the Specific

   You will deny any other method UNTIL the clinician asks about a gun:

   1. **Have owned a gun for protection for years**
   2. **Five weeks ago, while drinking at night, you took the gun and drove to a field in an isolated section of countryside**
   3. **While in the field you loaded the gun**
   4. **Clicked safety off**
   5. **Placed gun up against temple, placing it up and down about 5 times**
   6. **Decided you could not shoot yourself, once again because, "I can't do this to the kids"**
   7. **Gun is kept, "Where I can get it if I need it"**

If the clinician uses the Catch-All Question, "Are there any other ways you've thought of killing yourself that we haven't talked about?"

   Simply say "No."

Clinician will use Symptom Amplification

   You will say, "Not all the time, I don't know, maybe 60% of the day."

Tips for Role-Player:

1. As the clinician uses behavioral incidents to make any verbal videos, progressively share the many steps you've taken **(but only provide a step or two at a time of your actions, because you want the interviewer to learn how to use a series of behavioral incidents)**

Index

Note: Page numbers of article titles are in **boldface** type.

Psychiatr Clin N Am 38 (2015) 185–192
http://dx.doi.org/10.1016/S0193-953X(15)00011-8
0193-953X/15/$ – see front matter

Moving?

Make sure your subscription moves with you!

To notify us of your new address, find your **Clinics Account Number** (located on your mailing label above your name), and contact customer service at:

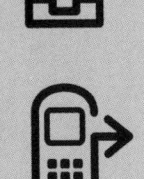

Email: **journalscustomerservice-usa@elsevier.com**

800-654-2452 (subscribers in the U.S. & Canada)
314-447-8871 (subscribers outside of the U.S. & Canada)

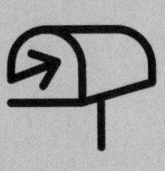

Fax number: **314-447-8029**

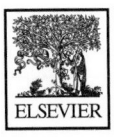

Elsevier Health Sciences Division
Subscription Customer Service
3251 Riverport Lane
Maryland Heights, MO 63043

*To ensure uninterrupted delivery of your subscription, please notify us at least 4 weeks in advance of move.